MAKER'S DIET
Meals

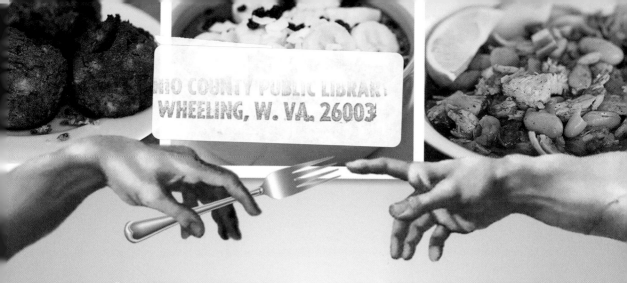

MAKER'S DIET
Meals

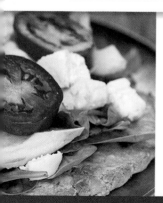
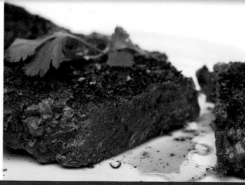
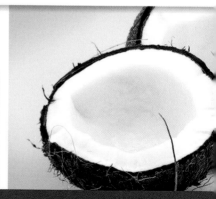

JORDAN RUBIN
WITH DR. JOSH AXE & DEB WILLIAMS

Destiny Image® Publishers, Inc.
P.O. Box 310, Shippensburg, PA
17257-0310

"Promoting Inspired Lives"

Recipes: Jordan and Nicki Rubin, Josh Axe, Deb Williams, Kelcie Yeo, Kate Battistelli
Editors, Managers, Designers: Evan Tardy, Carrie Medeiros
Photographer: David Molnar

This book and all other Destiny Image and Destiny Image Fiction books are available at Christian bookstores and distributors worldwide.

For more information on foreign distributors, call 717-532-3040.

Reach us on the Internet:
www.destinyimage.com

ISBN 13 HC: 978-0-7684-4231-1
ISBN 13 TP: 978-0-7684-0687-0
ISBN Ebook: 978-0-7684-8469-4

For Worldwide Distribution, Printed in the U.S.A.

1 2 3 4 5 6 7 / 18 17 16 15 14

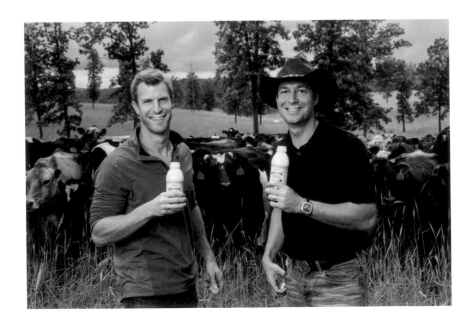

A special thank you to Kelcie Yeo and Kate Battistelli for all their hard work in making this cookbook come together, their amazing recipe contributions, and countless experiments in the kitchen perfecting each of these recipes.

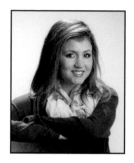

After suffering from chronic illnesses throughout her childhood, Kelcie Yeo found hope for healing by applying biblical principles to her diet. By eating food the way God intended for her to eat, she became well. Kelcie completed the Beyond Organic University Health Coach certification program in 2012. Her blog, www.kelcieskreations.blogspot.com, provides recipes for those who want to enjoy healthy food that tastes great! Her mission is to help people change their diet, change their life, and together take back the dominion of biblical principles in the areas of health and wholeness.

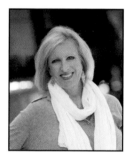

Kate Battistelli is a blogger and the author of *Growing Great Kids: Partner with God to Cultivate His Purpose in Your Child's Life*, published by Charisma House. She's currently working on her second book, *The God Dare,* to be released this fall. She's been married for 31 years to her husband, Mike, and she's the mom of recording artist Francesca Battistelli. She blogs about food, family, hospitality, and faith at KateBattistelli.com. You can find her on Twitter, Instagram, and Facebook.

table of contents

main dishes

salads

side dishes

snacks

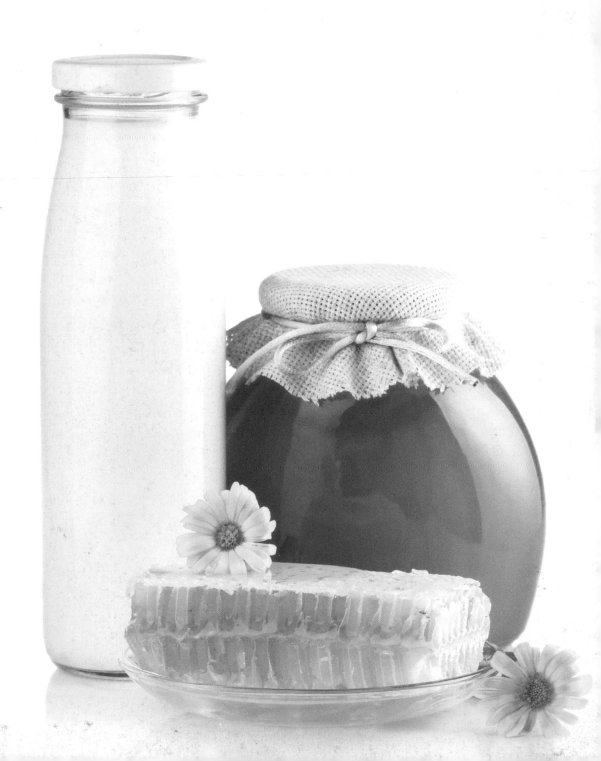

maker's diet
meals

If you want to experience incredible health in body, mind, and spirit, then it's time to heed the nutritional wisdom of the Bible.

Maker's Diet Meals helps you put into practice ancient nutritional principles that biblical heroes like Abraham, Isaac, Jacob, Moses, Daniel, David, and even our savior Jesus lived thousands of years ago.

The focus of this cookbook is not counting calories, fat, or carbs, and we are not going to make you eat sticks and grass, or locusts and honey for that matter, even though we think that raw honey can make just about anything taste great!

Maker's Diet Meals follows God's dietary principles and focuses on helping you consume the most nutrient-dense superfoods in the world to help you reach your full God-given health potential.

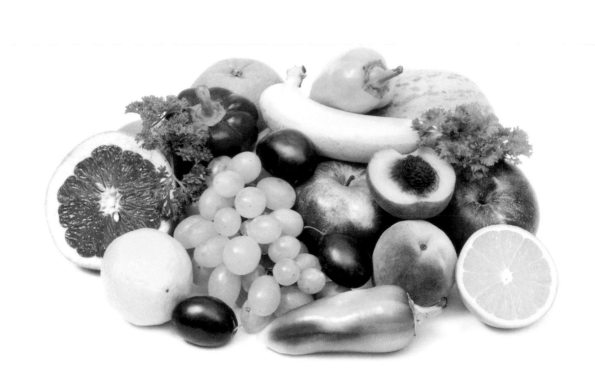

Why Maker's Diet?

Before we show you exactly *what* to eat, let's talk about *why* following a biblical way of eating can transform your health. A great place to start is in the book of Daniel. In Daniel chapter one we read the account of four young men of God—Daniel, Hananiah, Mishael, and Azariah—who refused to eat the king's delicacies (junk food).

They were avoiding the king's foods because in doing so they would defile themselves according to God's commandments as the meats served were likely detestable—sacrificed to idols, strangled, containing fatty portions, and with blood left in them. Daniel requested that they only be given "pulse" (basically vegetables, fruits, nuts, and seeds) and water, and then be tested to see the results of their Maker's recommended diet.

10 days later...

Daniel and his friends were healthier and stronger than all of the other young men training for the king's council.

3 years later...

Upon examination by the king, Daniel, Hananiah, Mishael, and Azariah were found to be ten times greater in wisdom and understanding than all the other young men of their age. Imagine that, ten times greater! God had given Daniel, Hananiah, Mishael, and Azariah knowledge and skill in all things and the king found none like them in matters of wisdom and understanding in all his kingdom. Also, Daniel went on to outlive King Nebuchadnezzar and actually counsel a third successive king roughly 70 years later!

One of the most important aspects about Daniel's diet was not just what he ate, but why he ate it. He did it to honor God. I believe that is the main reason he saw supernatural results and favor in his life.

While Daniel chose to eat only plant based foods during his 10-day diet, I don't believe he was a vegetarian all of his life. In fact, when you study the diet of the fathers of our faith you see that Abraham, Moses, David, and even Jesus consumed healthy animal foods such as meat and dairy, but only that which was raised and cared for by God's standards. These men consumed a diet rich in wild and pasture-raised meats, cultured dairy, vegetables, fruits, nuts, and seeds with many living 100-plus years in vibrant health.

I think the apostle Paul sums up the Maker's Diet mindset best in 1 Corinthians 10:31:

"WHETHER YOU EAT, DRINK, OR WHATEVER YOU DO, DO IT ALL FOR THE GLORY OF GOD."

Maker's Diet Plate

For years Americans followed the nutrition advice of the USDA's Food Pyramid that recommended you consume six to eleven servings of grains a day. The American people have followed that advice and are now paying dearly for it with their bulging waistlines and lack of vitality!

In more recent years, the recommendations have changed from a pyramid and taken the form of a plate. Even though there are improvements in their recommendations, they still have many flaws.

So what's the solution? The Maker's Plate! This can give you a blueprint of what your ideal meals can look like when you are striving for a healthy diet. Your plate should be full of nutrient-dense foods such as vegetables, fruits, nuts, seeds, pasture-raised meat and poultry, wild-caught fish, and cultured dairy.

Vegetables and Fruits / Meat and Dairy / Sprouted Nuts / Seeds / Grains / Glass of Spring Water

top lists 10

If you want to honor God with your body, then we recommend you not focus just on calories in the foods you eat but rather on the nutrients the food provides. You want to eat a nutrient-dense diet that is packed with vitamins and minerals as well as beneficial compounds such as enzymes, antioxidants, probiotics, and organic acids. Here are the top 10 lists for Probiotic, Antioxidant, and Metabolism boosting foods.

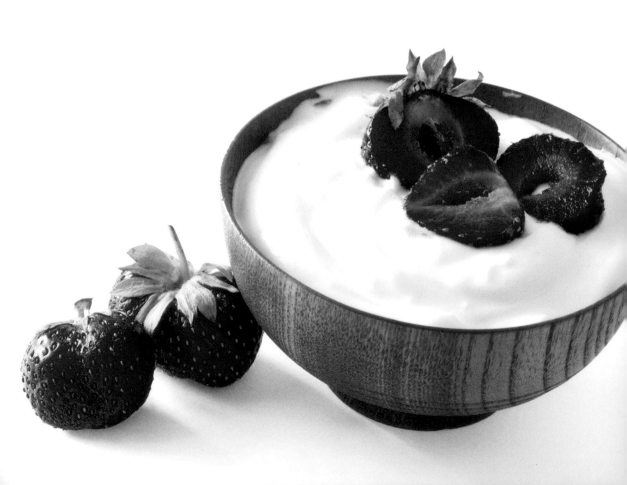

Probiotics Are Powerful

Probiotics are good germs that line your digestive tract and support your body's ability to absorb nutrients and protect your health. There are actually ten times more probiotics in your gut then cells in your body! Probiotics have been proven effective in supporting immune function and healthy digestion, as well as beautiful skin.

Most people are in need of a probiotic boost due to the use of prescription medication, particularly antibiotics, as well as a high sugar diet, and the consumption of chlorinated water and conventional foods such as non-organic meat, dairy, and eggs which contain antibiotic residues.

Top 10 Probiotics

1. Amasai	6. Kvass
2. Fermented Herbs and Spices	7. Natto
3. Cultured Whey	8. Yogurt (goat or sheep milk)
4. Cultured Vegetables	9. Raw Cheese (A1 beta casein free)
5. Kombucha	10. Keflr (goat milk)

We've all heard the principle you are what you eat, but really you are what you digest. And there are no other compounds in the world that support digestion and the assimilation of nutrients better than living probiotics.

The world's healthiest people in every corner of our planet have consumed probiotic rich foods with virtually every meal, and we believe you should too. Also, it's good to receive a wide variety of probiotic species in your diet to provide ultimate digestive support.

Amazing Antioxidants

Antioxidants are compounds that protect your cells from oxidation. Oxidation is the same process that browns an apple or rusts metal.

When antioxidant levels in the body are lower than they should be due to poor nutrition, the resulting oxidation can damage cells which can cause you to age at an accelerated rate. There are some foods that contain high levels of antioxidants and others that cause your body to produce antioxidants such as glutathione. Some of the best known antioxidants are polyphenols, carotenoids, and vitamins A, C, and E.

Top 10 Antioxidant Food and Beverages

1. **Berries:** *blueberry, raspberry, blackberry, strawberry*	6. **Teas:** *white, green, black, and rooibos*
2. **Kale**	7. **Red Cabbage**
3. **Turmeric**	8. **Wild Salmon**
4. **Pomegranate**	9. **Coffee**
5. **Cinnamon**	10. **Raw Chocolate (Cacao)**

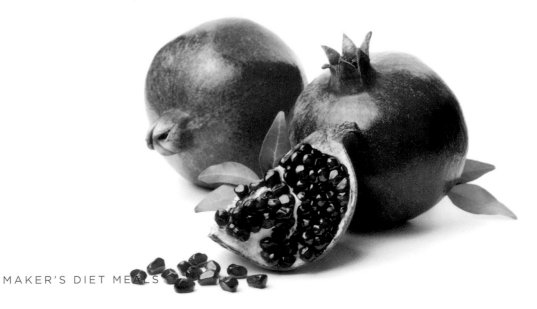

Master Your Metabolism

If you want to burn excess body fat, exercise isn't the only way to go. Consuming certain foods can rev up your metabolism and help you reach your ideal weight.

Top 10 Metabolism Boosting Foods

1. Chia Seeds	**6. Seaweed**
2. Tea: *black, green, white, oolong, rooibos*	**7. Berries**
3. Green Leafy Vegetables	**8. Raw Cheese** *(free of beta casein A1)*
4. Pasture-Raised Beef	**9. Coffee**
5. Coconut *(meat, oil, fiber)*	**10. Cultured Vegetables**

Some of the key factors for supporting a healthy metabolism are fatty acids such as MCFAs (medium chain fatty acids), SCFAs (short chain fatty acids), omega-3, and CLA. Amino acids are critical for building muscle. Surprisingly, your best sources of these nutrients are meat and dairy.

Fiber plays an important role in keeping your body fit and your stomach full. Nuts, seeds, legumes, fruits, and vegetables provide all that you need in the fiber category. And last but not least, there are certain phytonutrients found in foods such as polyphenols and flavanoids that can keep your metabolism running smoothly.

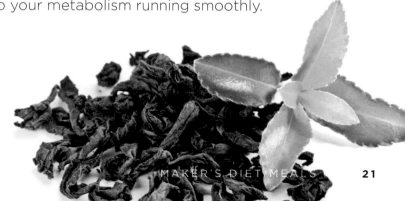

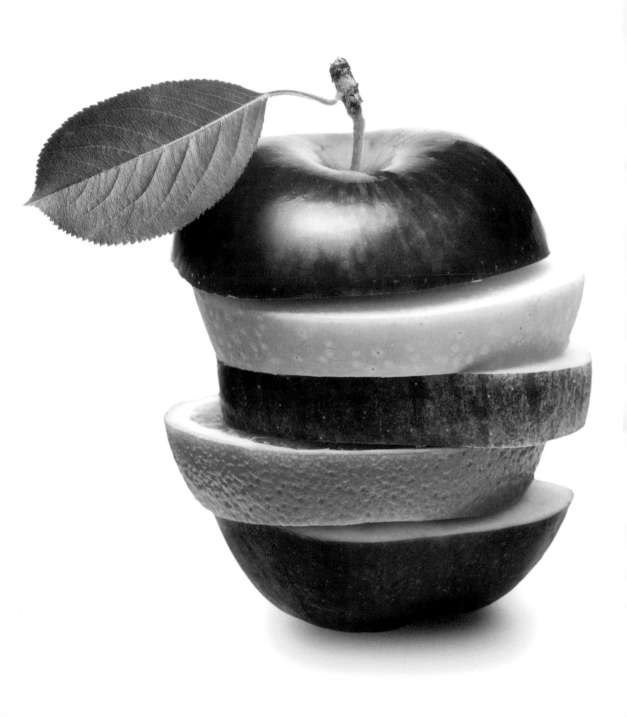

maker's diet
standards

When it comes to eating God's way, the following standards serve as a great place to start.

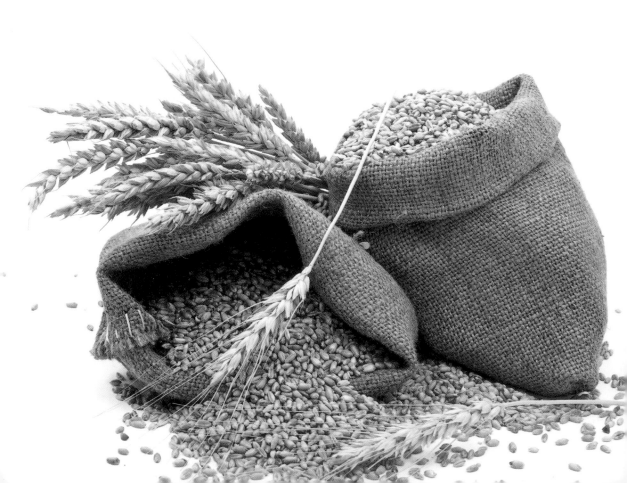

1. Say No to GMO

Genetically modified foods containing genetically modified organisms (GMO) are just what the name implies. They are foods that have been genetically altered and have moved away from God's original design.

GM foods have altered genetic codes by wiring in genes from other forms of life, including other plants, pesticides, bacteria, and viruses. Most GM foods today have been modified to tolerate or even produce pesticides. It is believed that GMOs can contribute to many health challenges and the long-term risks could be much greater than we can even imagine.

More and more foods are becoming genetically modified, but the most common are corn, soybeans, canola, cotton seeds, zucchini, summer squash, alfalfa, papaya, and sugar beets. Unless these foods are specifically labeled as organic or GMO free, you may be better off assuming they are genetically modified.

2. Avoid Gluten

While the grains found in biblical times were undoubtedly healthy, with today's mass hybridization, the gluten containing grains (wheat, barley, rye) are causing many health problems.

> ## Gluten is the sticky protein found in wheat, barley, rye, and some oat products.

Gluten causes health issues for many people and according to the NIDDK, Celiac disease affects 1 in 133 Americans. However, as many as one in five people are gluten intolerant and I believe the majority of Americans do not digest gluten containing grains efficiently. Some common symptoms of gluten intolerance include bloating, anxiety, behavior issues in children, joint pain, malabsorption, poor thyroid function, fatigue, and weight gain.

The bulk of our dietary gluten consumption is found in wheat products today. Wheat is a highly hybridized crop and these modern farming methods have been used to grow wheat that is fungal resistant and produces a higher yield, but is also much lower in nutrients and higher in gluten.

Not all wheat products are necessarily unhealthy. There are more desirable strains that are non-hybridized and grow wild like kamut and einkorn wheat. We also believe if you are going to consume grain products they are best sprouted or sour leavened. The process of sprouting or sour leavening breaks down the gluten components, allowing many to more easily digest grains in these forms.

3. Say No to the "Devil in the Milk"

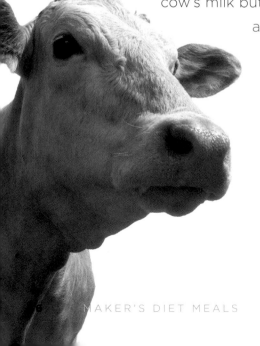

Have you ever wondered why someone could be sensitive to cow's milk but not goat's milk? Or have you ever thought about how an infant could do great on its mother's milk but when given cow's milk could not tolerate it?

Human breast milk as well as the milk from ruminant animals such as cows, sheep, and goats contain two types of protein—whey and casein.

But according to new research from Dr. Keith Woodford, not all casein is created equal. All human milk, sheep, and goat's milk is free of A1 beta casein and contains A2 casein. Nearly all cow's milk dairy in America—whether raw or pasteurized, organic or conventional—contains A1 beta casein.

It is believed that the A1 casein, which is a foreign protein to humans, is the cause of much of the dairy intolerance we're experiencing today. In fact, the presence of A1 beta casein in dairy might make it significantly more problematic for our health than gluten.

Dairy is great when it's sourced from cows exclusively fed on pasture and cultured with powerful probiotics. In fact, the right kind of dairy can perhaps be considered the perfect food. Dairy has been consumed for thousands of years and some of the longest lived people in the world have subsisted mostly on dairy, including our biblical ancestors. According to Dr. Keith Woodford, in his book *Devil in the Milk,* sometime in the past 2,000 years a genetic mutation has occurred which caused one species of cattle (Bos taurus) to produce A1 casein.

The original species of cattle from India, Africa, and the Middle East produces milk free of A1 beta casein. This type of cow is known as a Zebu (Bos indicus). We call milk that is free of A1 beta casein Z-Milk in honor of the Zebu cattle that originally produce it. Z-milk has a protein structure that more closely resembles human breast milk. Cultured, green-fed, organic Z-milk is easy to digest and has advantages over goat and sheep milk.

4. No Chemicals (Pesticides, Herbicides, or Fungicides)

If you saw someone pull out a sprayer and douse an apple with pesticides, then hand it to you and say, "Have a bite"—would you eat it? Probably not. Our grocery stores today offer mostly conventional produce that has been grown with chemical fertilizers and sprayed with chemicals as well.

Pesticides will not kill you by consuming just one apple that has been sprayed. The problem occurs when you consume these foods over time and the toxins accumulate in your cells and organs. Pesticides and herbicides in our food supply have been linked to an increase in toxicity and many health challenges.

5. No Hormones, Antibiotics, or Vaccines

According to research out of the *Journal of Agriculture and Food Chemistry,* scientists have detected an average of 21 different chemicals and medications found in your milk and meat supply, including:

Growth Hormones	Painkillers
Steroids	Anti-Inflammatory Medications
Antibiotic Drugs	Birth Control Pills
Anti-Fungal Drugs	Heart Medications

Recently, the American Cancer Society stated that recombinant bovine growth hormone (rBGH) is just one of the synthetic (man-made) hormones given to our cows to increase milk production. Unfortunately, it has been proven to harm the animals and increase human levels of IGF-1 which may promote unhealthy cell growth in humans.

We know that dairy and meat products are wonderful sources of nutrients if they are raised and processed using biblical standards. There are few foods in the world that have the combination of omega-3 fats, probiotics, and bone and muscle building nutrients as healthy dairy.

6. No High Heat Processing

Over the last decade we have seen the debate over raw foods versus cooked foods elevate, especially in the dairy category. Pasteurization and homogenization can denature proteins and destroy nutrients. High heat processing can destroy enzymes like phosphatase, which is important for bone health, and lactase, which supports digestion. Many vitamins are also impacted, including B vitamins.

Today, pasteurization extends beyond dairy to many other foods and beverages. Everything from fruit juice to shelled nuts such as almonds are subjected to high heat. Every day more foods are pasteurized in an attempt to make up for unsanitary conditions, but high heat processing that destroys beneficial bacteria and other essential nutrients may cause more harm than good.

When buying any food product, we recommend you stay away from ultra-high temperature pasteurization, which heats the product as high as 185-260 degrees, and instead look for raw foods or, in the case of dairy, low temperature pasteurized.

7. Biblically Based Land Management and Animal Slaughter Methods

In the book of Leviticus, God gives food laws advising us to stay away from animals that are carriers of toxins such as pigs and shellfish, along with commands on giving the land a Sabbath rest every seventh year. There are also strict commandments ensuring proper slaughter methods for animals the Bible considers fit for human consumption.

In Leviticus 25:4 God says, "In the seventh year the land must have a Sabbath year of complete rest. Do not sow your fields or prune your vineyards during that year."

This wisdom of God allows the soil to replenish its nutrients and keeps the land healthy. Today, in modern agriculture, we do not let the soil rest and rarely rotate our crops. This causes the soil to become depleted of nutrients, and then typically only three synthetic minerals are added back—nitrogen, potassium, and phosphorus.

Most animals today are slaughtered in one of four ways—electrocution, gassing, head trauma, or the shotgun method. When animals aren't slaughtered using the biblical or kosher methods it can send a surge of stress hormones through their system, which can lead to additional health problems when humans consume their meat. So make sure you buy meat products from a company that uses biblically based methods of slaughter.

8. Go Grass-Fed

We've all heard the principle "you are what you eat," but when you eat animal foods, you are what *they* ate. When cattle consume grains such as corn it disrupts the ratio of omega-6 to omega-3 fatty acids in the meat. In turn, the increase in omega-6 fats can lead to imbalances in the body. That's why you should only consume beef and dairy products that have been fed exclusively on green foods or what is known as grass-fed.

Animals that are pasture-raised on grasses, legumes, forbs, and herbs year round have high levels of omega-3 fats and CLA—an important fatty acid.

According to California State University, pasture-fed beef contains three times as much CLA (conjugated linoleic acid) than grain-fed beef. According to the *American Journal of Clinical Nutrition,* CLA has been studied to boost your metabolism and support cellular health.

9. Nothing Artificial

There couldn't be anything further from real food than artificial sweeteners such as aspartame. Aspartame has been linked to 92 adverse health effects, including headaches, memory loss, and anxiety. Aspartame breaks down into phenylalanine, aspartic acid, and methanol, which eventually breaks down into a substance resembling formaldehyde.

Sucralose is another common artificial sweetener that is 600 times sweeter than table sugar.

Chlorinated compounds such as sucralose have been found to stockpile in your intestinal tract, kidneys, and liver causing toxicity over time. So now you may be wondering what you can do to satisfy your sweet tooth? The next section has some suggestions we think you'll find to be sweet!

Satisfy Your Sweet Tooth

There are several natural sweeteners that can be used in place of refined sugar. Our favorites include raw honey, coconut nectar, maple syrup, and whole green leaf stevia. That being said, we still recommend sweeteners be used in moderation. Here are some details about our favorite natural sweeteners.

Raw Honey

Throughout history honey has been an important food. God used honey to motivate the Israelite people when He told them, "Go up to the land flowing with milk and honey" (Exodus 33:3).

Honey is far more than a sweetener; it can even be called a "functional food." Raw honey contains enzymes, amino acids, antioxidants, B vitamins, and trace minerals. Raw honey aids in digestive health and does not ferment in the digestive tract like most other sources of sugar. It has anti-microbial properties and has even historically been used topically on wounds. When buying honey try and find local raw honey.

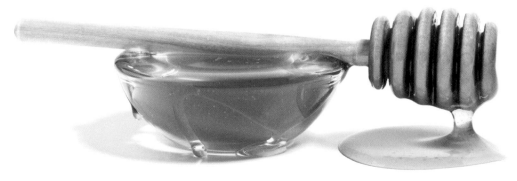

According to research, 70 percent of store bought honey contains no pollen and really shouldn't be called honey at all. Check your local health food store and farmers market for the best available honey.

Coconut Sugar

Coconut sugar or nectar is the sap that comes from coconut blossoms. It is low on the glycemic index and contains 17 amino acids, minerals, and B vitamins. Coconut nectar can be used in baking and has a more neutral taste than most natural sweeteners.

Maple Syrup

When buying maple syrup, we recommend you buy grade B organic maple syrup because it is the least processed. Maple syrup contains malic acid which can be good for the digestive system and provides zinc and manganese.

Stevia

Stevia is a great natural sweetener and is best used in its whole green leaf form as opposed to the more common white processed version. The body does not metabolize the sweet glycosides from the stevia leaf, so there is no caloric intake. Stevia blends well in teas and snack foods and is a great alternative to those toxic artificial sweeteners.

Fat Is Fabulous

Fat has been given a pretty bad rap over the years and we want to dispel some of those myths. First, eating fat doesn't make you fat, but eating the wrong type of fat can make you unhealthy. Eating good fats can actually help you burn fat and lose weight! Below is a list of the most fabulous fats.

Extra Virgin Coconut Oil

Coconut oil is unique in that it is high in saturated fats but very good for you. Yeah, that's right, we said saturated fat. Saturated fats are essential to your health and longevity because they support your cell membrane flexibility and digestive health.

The predominant fatty type of fatty acids found in coconut are called medium chain fatty acids or MCFAs. MCFAs are not nine calories like most lipids but are eight calories and your body will burn this type of fat very efficiently.

There are many fitness programs today that promote the use of coconut oil as a natural fat burner and recommend it be used in place of other fats. Athletes and triathletes have started using coconut as a preferred fuel source because the body can easily use MCFAs for energy. Coconut oil has a high heat threshold so it's the ideal fat for cooking, frying, and baking.

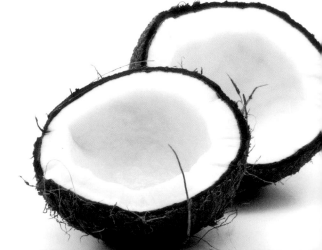

Real Butter Is Better

One of the healthiest foods you can consume in your diet is organic butter from pasture-raised cows. There was a time when many people turned away from butter and started consuming margarine, but now we know that the hydrogenated fats in margarine can lead to poor health.

Butter contains two important fats that can help bring your health to the next level. Short chain fatty acids (SCFAs) found in butter provide great health benefits. Butyric acid or butyrate has been shown to support growth of good bacteria and support healthy inflammation levels in the gut.

Another healthy fat found in butter is conjugated linoleic acid (CLA). CLA has been demonstrated to support healthy metabolism.

It's essential when buying butter or any dairy product that it comes exclusively from pasture-fed animals.

Extra Virgin Olive Oil

Most of us have heard over the years that olive is the healthiest oil. Extra virgin olive oil is wonderful, but we recommend you *not* cook with it. When olive oil is heated over 250 degrees, the oil can oxidize, creating free radicals, and the high heat destroys some of the oil's delicate nutrients and beneficial compounds.

So do we still recommend using olive oil? Absolutely! Just not for cooking. Use it in salad dressings, homemade sauces, and drizzle it on your favorite dishes.

Olive oil is high in omega-9 monounsaturated fatty acids that have been proven to support heart health. Also, when buying olive oil, always buy organic extra virgin olive oil.

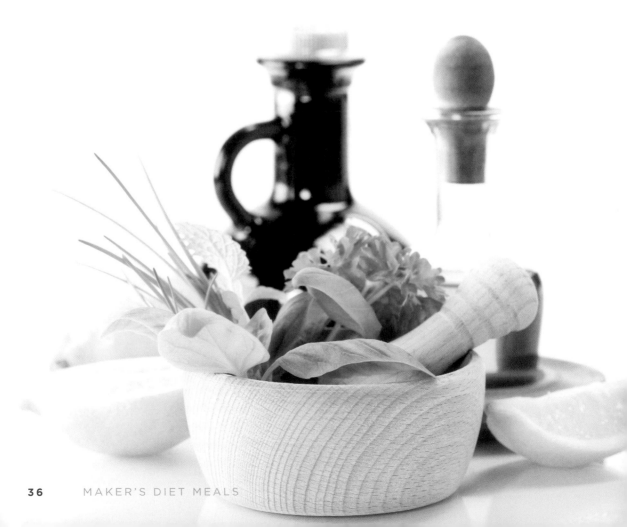

Is *Maker's Diet Meals* Organic?

Many people wonder if organic food is truly better than conventional. Absolutely! But are all organic foods healthy? Not necessarily. Many organic foods can be found lining the aisles of health food stores that are loaded with sugar, unhealthy fats, white flour, and processed ingredients.

That's why *Maker's Diet Meals* goes *beyond* organic and only includes foods that are grown, raised, and processed to the highest available standard—the biblical standard.

If you are shopping on a budget and wondering what the most important foods to buy organic would be, below are lists known as the Toxic Two, Dirty Dozen, and the Clean Fifteen.

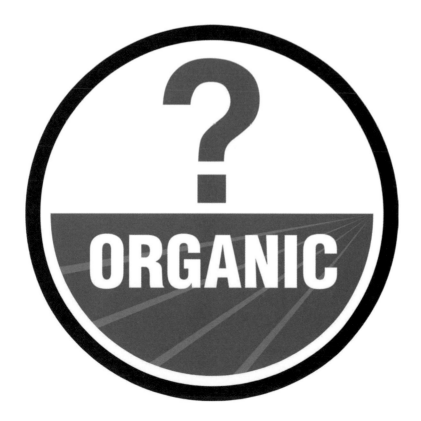

The Toxic Two

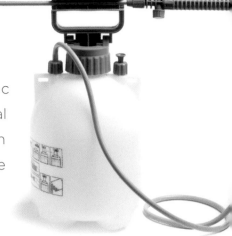

Even more important than choosing organic produce, organic meat and dairy are critical as their conventional counterparts can contain toxins stored in their fat. Also, we recommend staying away from pork, farm-raised fish, and shellfish.

Conventional Meat
Conventional Dairy

Instead, replace these conventional products with organic, 100 percent grass-fed beef, wild-caught fish, pastured eggs and poultry, green-fed dairy, and wild game.

The Dirty Dozen

The fruits and vegetables that rank the highest in pesticide load are known as the Dirty Dozen, and the Environmental Working Group advises that if you can't afford to buy all organic produce, you should at least buy organic versions of these 12 items. A good rule of thumb is if you consume the outer layer or the peel, it's more important to buy organic.

Apples	Peaches	Cucumbers
Strawberries	Green Leafy	Potatoes
Grapes	Vegetables	Cherry
Celery	Bell Peppers	Tomatoes
	Nectarines	Hot Peppers

The Clean Fifteen

The produce on this list contain the least amount of pesticide contamination and are known as the Clean Fifteen. In general, foods where you do not eat the outside or the peel have lower levels of pesticides.

Mushrooms	Eggplant	Cabbage
Sweet	Asparagus	Avocados
Potatoes	Mangos	Pineapple
Cantaloupe	Papayas	Onions
Grapefruit	Sweet Peas	Corn
Kiwi		

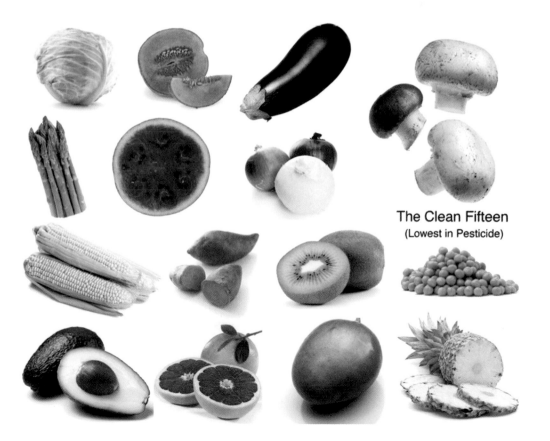

The Clean Fifteen
(Lowest in Pesticide)

Biblical Fermentation

Question: What is the difference between:

Apple Juice vs. Apple Cider Vinegar

Regular Bread vs. Ezekiel Bread

Cabbage vs. Sauerkraut

Milk vs. Yogurt

The answer—fermentation. Fermentation is a process that breaks down substances, making them more readily absorbed. Fermentation literally unlocks the nutrients inside the food and creates entirely new and beneficial compounds as well!

When it comes to grains, legumes, nuts, and seeds, fermentation can disarm anti-nutrients of their mineral blocking power.

For instance, even though cabbage has many vitamins and minerals, when you take cabbage and ferment it into sauerkraut, it creates higher levels of vitamin C, B vitamins, enzymes, probiotics, and four new sulphur compounds that may have amazing health boosting benefits! So load up on fermented foods such as cultured dairy, apple cider vinegar, and fermented living herbals. Fermenting your own foods can take time but the health benefits are unparalleled.

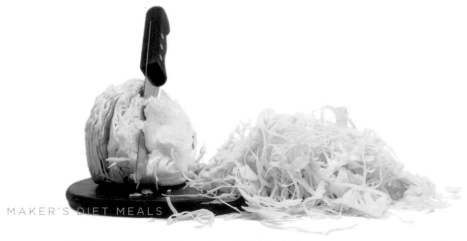

food
SWITCHES

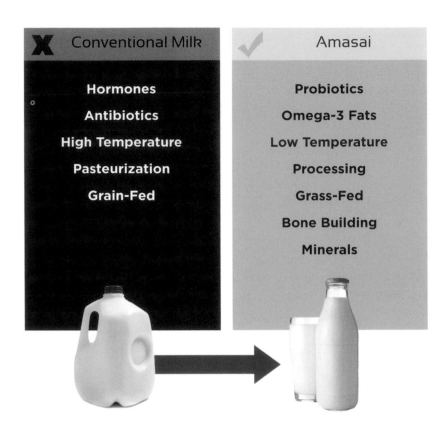

✗ Conventional Milk	✓ Amasai
Hormones	Probiotics
Antibiotics	Omega-3 Fats
High Temperature	Low Temperature
Pasteurization	Processing
Grain-Fed	Grass-Fed
	Bone Building
	Minerals

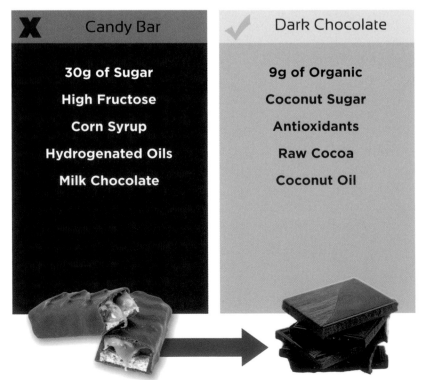

✗ Candy Bar	✓ Dark Chocolate
30g of Sugar	9g of Organic
High Fructose	Coconut Sugar
Corn Syrup	Antioxidants
Hydrogenated Oils	Raw Cocoa
Milk Chocolate	Coconut Oil

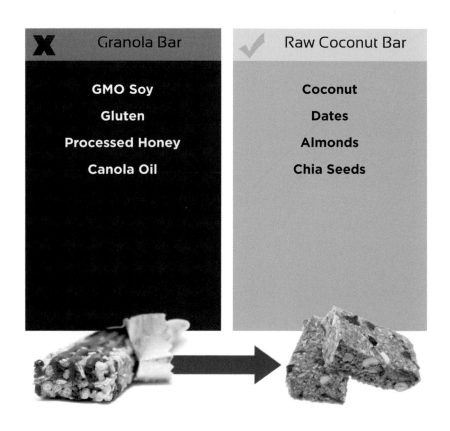

✗ Granola Bar	✓ Raw Coconut Bar
GMO Soy	**Coconut**
Gluten	**Dates**
Processed Honey	**Almonds**
Canola Oil	**Chia Seeds**

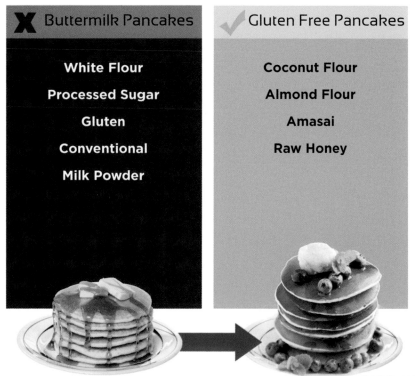

✗ Buttermilk Pancakes	✓ Gluten Free Pancakes
White Flour	**Coconut Flour**
Processed Sugar	**Almond Flour**
Gluten	**Amasai**
Conventional Milk Powder	**Raw Honey**

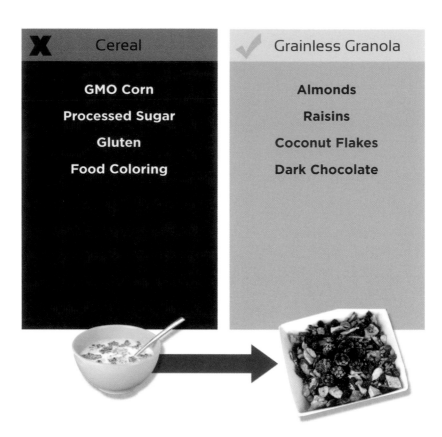

✗ Cereal	✓ Grainless Granola
GMO Corn	Almonds
Processed Sugar	Raisins
Gluten	Coconut Flakes
Food Coloring	Dark Chocolate

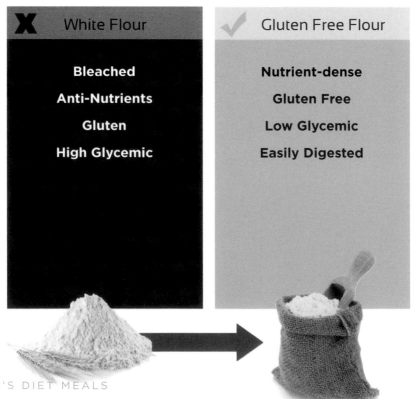

✗ White Flour	✓ Gluten Free Flour
Bleached	Nutrient-dense
Anti-Nutrients	Gluten Free
Gluten	Low Glycemic
High Glycemic	Easily Digested

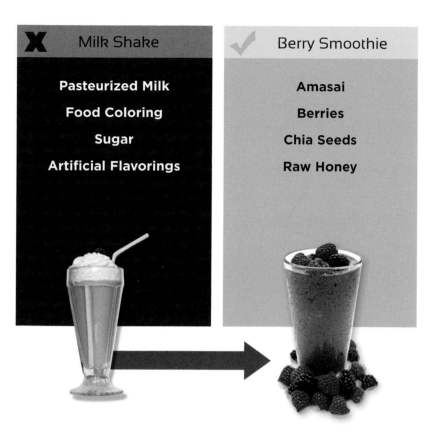

✗ Milk Shake	**✓ Berry Smoothie**
Pasteurized Milk	**Amasai**
Food Coloring	**Berries**
Sugar	**Chia Seeds**
Artificial Flavorings	**Raw Honey**

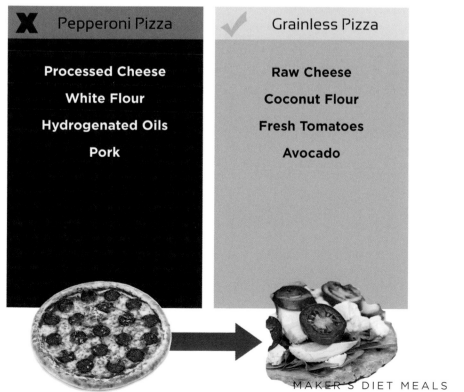

✗ Pepperoni Pizza	**✓ Grainless Pizza**
Processed Cheese	**Raw Cheese**
White Flour	**Coconut Flour**
Hydrogenated Oils	**Fresh Tomatoes**
Pork	**Avocado**

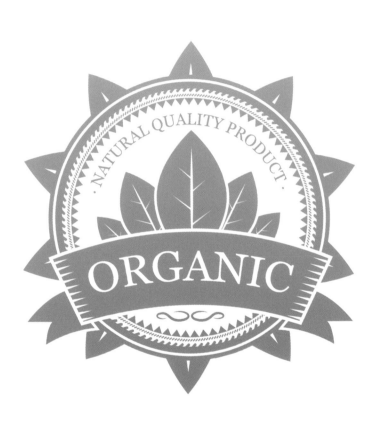

important
message

Important Message: We believe that consuming organic foods is a healthy way to live. Based on that belief, all of the recipes in *Maker's Diet Meals* are best made using organic ingredients. Therefore, we do not use the term "organic" before each ingredient in the recipes as the organic nature is assumed.

Several ingredients listed as optional such as Terrain Living Herbals, cultured whey, green-fed cheeses, and Amasai are available at www.livebeyondorganic.com.

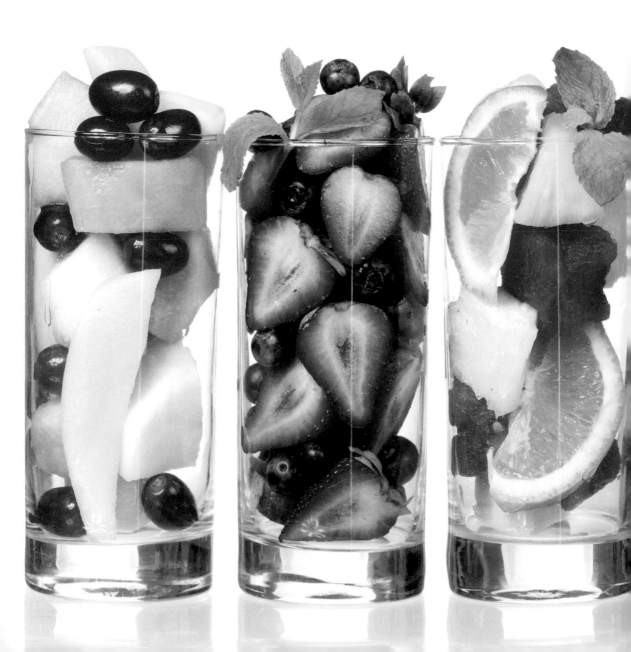

beverages

AVOCADO SMOOTHIE

Avocado Smoothie

2 really ripe bananas

½ avocado

8 oz plain Amasai or coconut milk

2 Tbsp ground chia seeds

1 tsp vanilla

2 cups kale/spinach

1 cup ice

> Blend in blender until rich and creamy.

> Makes two 8-ounce servings.

Orange Cream Smoothie

8 oz of plain Amasai or sheep milk yogurt

4 oz freshly squeezed orange juice

1-2 raw, pastured eggs (optional)

1-2 Tbsp raw, unheated honey

1-2 fresh or frozen bananas

¼ tsp vanilla extract

> Combine the ingredients in a high–speed blender.

> Makes two 8-ounce servings.

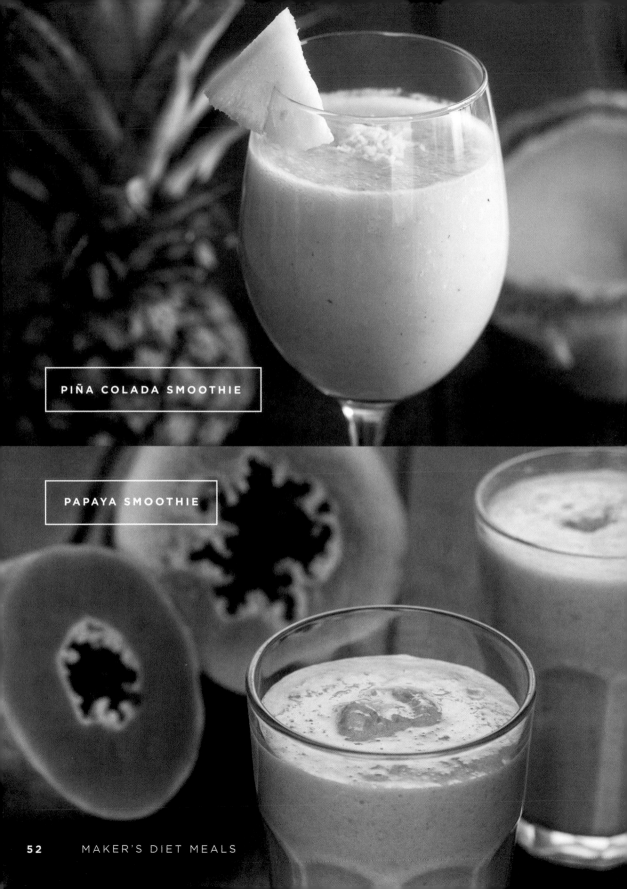

PIÑA COLADA SMOOTHIE

PAPAYA SMOOTHIE

Piña Colada Smoothie

10 oz of plain Amasai or coconut milk

1-2 raw, pastured eggs (optional)

1 Tbsp extra virgin coconut oil

1-2 Tbsp raw, unheated honey

1 cup fresh or frozen pineapple

½ fresh or frozen banana

½ tsp vanilla extract

> Combine the ingredients in a high-speed blender.
> Makes two servings.

Papaya Smoothie

1 small papaya

1 ripe banana

8 oz plain Amasai

1 cup ice

> Blend in blender until creamy.

Raw Almond Milk

2 cups raw almonds

16 oz cultured whey

4 cups purified water

1 tsp vanilla extract

8 oz plain Amasai or coconut milk

1 cup ice

> Soak almonds overnight in cultured whey.
> Strain almonds and pour in blender.
> Add water and vanilla.
> Blend and strain through cheese cloth.
> Makes eight 8-ounce servings.

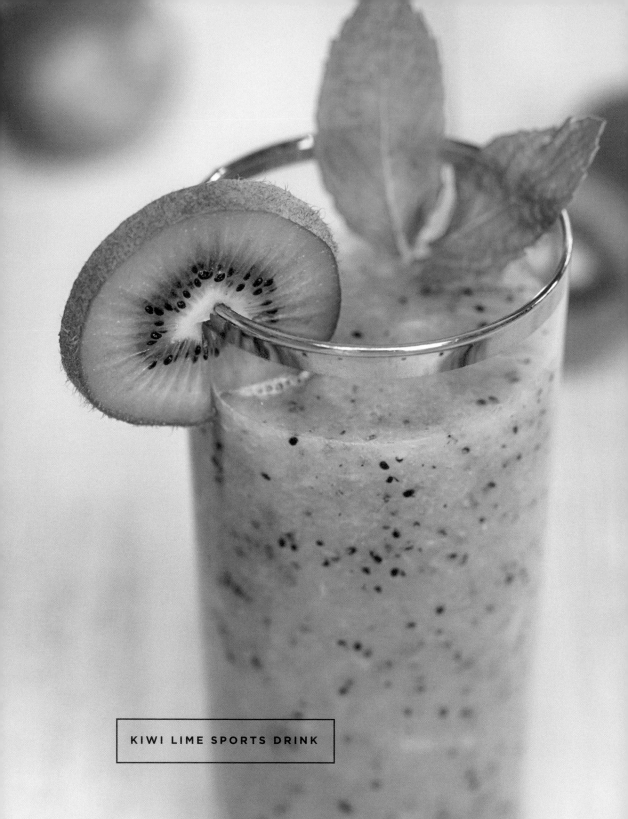

KIWI LIME SPORTS DRINK

Kiwi Lime Sports Drink

2 kiwis

Zest from 1 lime

Juice from 1 lime

8 oz cultured whey

1 Tbsp raw, unheated honey

1 cup ice

> Blend in blender until smooth and frothy.

> Makes two 8-ounce servings.

Berry Green Smoothie

1 cucumber, peeled

1 cup berries, fresh or frozen (blueberries, raspberries, blackberries, or cherries)

½ apple (with peel on)

3-4 leaves of kale

30 milliliters Terrain Ginger or Terrain Turmeric (optional)

½ lemon

1 avocado

> Cut the cucumber and apple in chunks. Place the cucumber, apple, and berries in a blender and process until smooth.

> Chop the greens and add to the blender along with the juice of half a lemon, the Terrain Ginger or Terrain Turmeric, and process until smooth. Add the avocado and process until well blended.

> Makes two servings.

Peaches and Cream Smoothie

10 oz plain Amasai or sheep milk yogurt

1-2 raw, pastured eggs (optional)

1-2 Tbsp raw, unheated honey

½-1 cup fresh or frozen peaches

1 fresh or frozen banana

½ tsp vanilla extract

> Combine the ingredients in a high-speed blender.

> Makes two 8-ounce servings.

Banana Cream Smoothie

10 oz of plain Amasai or sheep milk yogurt

1-2 raw, pastured eggs (optional)

1-2 Tbsp raw, unheated honey

1 cup fresh or frozen banana

½ tsp vanilla extract

3 Tbsp (1 serving) ground chia seeds

> Combine the ingredients in a high-speed blender.

> Makes two 8-ounce servings.

Swiss Almond Chocolate Smoothie

10 oz plain Amasai or coconut milk

1-2 raw, pastured eggs (optional)

1 Tbsp extra virgin coconut oil

1-2 Tbsp raw, unheated honey

2 Tbsp cocoa or cacao powder

2 Tbsp almond butter

1-2 fresh or frozen bananas

½ tsp vanilla extract

3 Tbsp ground chia seeds

> Combine the ingredients in a high-speed blender.

> Makes two 8-ounce servings.

Mochaccino Smoothie

10 oz plain Amasai or coconut milk

1-2 raw, pastured eggs (optional)

1 Tbsp extra virgin coconut oil

1-2 Tbsp raw, unheated honey

2 Tbsp cocoa or cacao powder

1 Tbsp whole coffee beans

1-2 fresh or frozen bananas

½ teaspoon vanilla extract

3 Tbsp ground chia seeds

> Combine the ingredients in a high-speed blender.

> Makes two servings.

breakfast

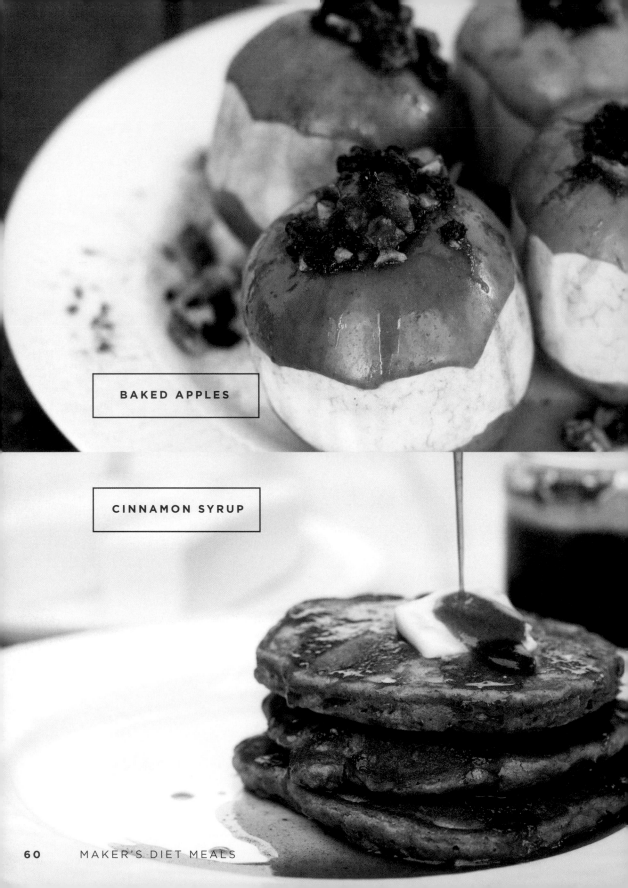

BAKED APPLES

CINNAMON SYRUP

Baked Apples

1 apple

1 tsp coconut sugar

1 Tbsp grass-fed butter

¼ tsp cinnamon

Dash nutmeg

1 Tbsp currants

1 Tbsp chopped pecans

1 Tbsp apple juice

1 tsp maple syrup

> Core apples and remove 1 inch of skin around middle. Mix butter, coconut sugar, cinnamon, nutmeg, currants, pecans, juice, and maple syrup together.

> Place apples upright in baking dish. Fill the centers of each apple with mixture. Pour hot water into baking pan until it is ¼ inch deep. Bake at 375 for 30-40 minutes.

> Drizzle the maple syrup over apples after they are done and return apples to the oven for another five minutes.

> Makes 1 baked apple.

Cinnamon Syrup

1 cup grade B maple syrup or raw, unheated honey

1 tsp cinnamon

¼ tsp mace or nutmeg

1 Tbsp butter

1 tsp vanilla

> In medium saucepan, over medium-high heat, whisk all ingredients together except the vanilla.

> Bring to a boil and boil for 1 minute.

> Take off heat and add vanilla.

VEGGIE OMELET

BUTTERNUT SQUASH PANCAKES

Veggie Omelet

3 pastured eggs

½ cup green-fed, raw cheddar cheese or goat cheese, shredded

1 large garlic clove

½ cup chopped red pepper

½ cup chopped green pepper

½ cup chopped mushroom

¼ cup chopped red onion

2 Tbsp grass-fed butter

> Sauté garlic, onion, peppers, mushrooms, and butter in the pan.
> After 5 minutes, add eggs.
> Shred the cheese on top and fold into an omelet.
> Serve with chives, oregano, and black pepper.
> Makes 1-2 servings.

Butternut Squash Pancakes

½ cup gluten-free flour

¾ tsp baking powder

¼ tsp baking soda

1 cup steamed butternut squash

¼ tsp salt

¾ tsp cinnamon

¼ tsp nutmeg

½ tsp ginger

½ cup Amasai

2 free range eggs

> Mix all ingredients together.
> Heat skillet on medium heat.
> Place 1 Tbsp coconut oil in skillet.
> Spoon out pancake batter into pan.
> Let them cook for approximately 5-7 minutes on each side.

MAPLE SAUSAGE PATTIES

Garden Frittata

3 Tbsp coconut oil

1 medium onion, chopped

1 small zucchini, chopped

1 small yellow squash, chopped

½ cup cherry tomatoes, cut in half

1 medium-sized red pepper, chopped

1 tsp sea salt

¼ tsp black pepper

1 tsp garlic powder

8 pastured eggs, beaten

½ cup green-fed, raw aged Havarti cheese, grated

2 Tbsp fresh parsley, chopped

2 Tbsp fresh basil, chopped

> In a medium oven-proof skillet, sauté the onions in the coconut oil until soft and transparent, over medium-high heat. Add chopped vegetables. Sauté until starting to soften.

> While squash mixture is sautéing, combine eggs, salt, pepper, cheese, parsley, and basil in a medium-sized bowl and stir well to combine all ingredients.

> Pour egg mixture over the vegetables in the skillet. Bake at 350 degrees for 35 minutes.

> Makes about 8 servings

Maple Sausage Patties

1 lb grass-fed ground beef

2 Tbsp coconut aminos

½ cup maple syrup

2 Tbsp coconut oil

> In large bowl, mix all ingredients together.

> In a large frying, pan place coconut oil and turn on at a low heat.

> Form meat into sausage patties and place in the pan.

> Cook with lid on for 15-20 minutes or until cooked!

> Serve with grain free pancakes and berries, or poached eggs and oranges.

> Serves 4.

SPINACH EGGS

CHOCOLATE CHIP BANANA BREAD

Spinach Eggs

6 cups firmly packed spinach leaves

2 Tbsp sun-dried tomatoes

1 shallot, chopped

2 Tbsp coconut oil

4 pastured eggs

1 oz green-fed raw cheddar cheese or goat cheese

1 tsp Italian seasoning

Sea salt and pepper to season

> In a medium skillet, heat the coconut oil and add shallot and cook for about 2 minutes over medium heat. Add spinach and cook for 3-4 minutes, stirring occasionally. Add sun-dried tomatoes and mix well.

> Distribute spinach/tomato mixture into ramekins.

> Crack one egg on top of each ramekin over spinach mixture. Season lightly with Italian seasoning and salt and pepper over each egg.

> Bake for about 15-18 minutes at 400 degrees. Remove from oven and sprinkle cheese over eggs.

> Serves 4.

Chocolate Chip Banana Bread

1 ripe banana

2 Tbsp coconut sugar

⅔ cup coconut oil

4 pastured eggs

1 tsp vanilla extract

½ cup coconut flour

1 tsp baking powder

½ cup dark chocolate chips

1 Tbsp sea salt

> Puree banana, coconut sugar, coconut oil, vanilla, and eggs together in a high-speed blender.

> Pour into a mixing bowl and add flour, salt, and baking powder.

> Fold in chocolate chips.

> Pour batter into a loaf pan and bake at 325 for 30 minutes.

> Serve with butter.

> Serves 4.

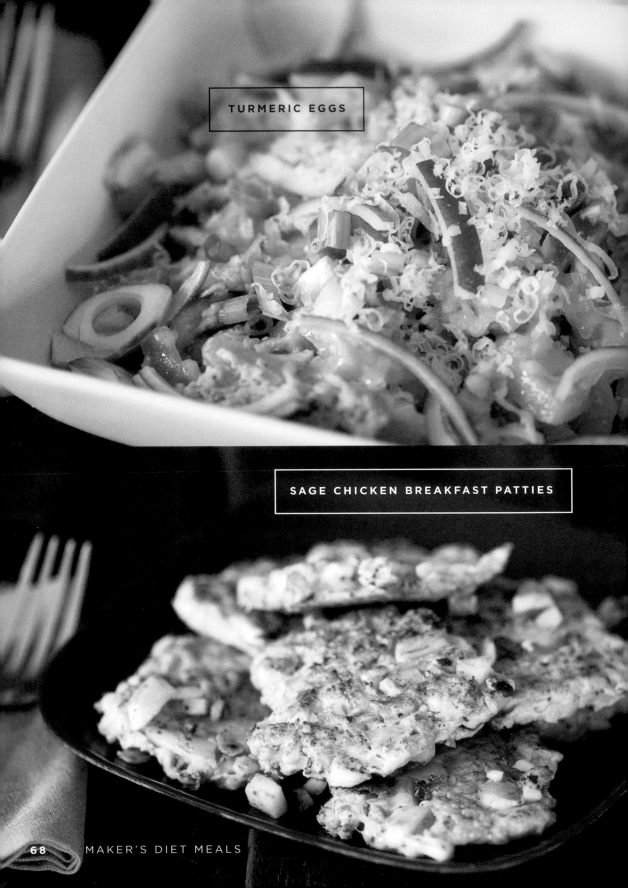

TURMERIC EGGS

SAGE CHICKEN BREAKFAST PATTIES

Turmeric Eggs

3 pastured eggs

2 oz shredded green-fed, raw cheddar cheese or goat cheese

3 Tbsp ghee

½ cup chopped red onions

8 chopped green onions

1 cup chopped yellow pepper

6 cloves minced garlic

1 Tbsp dried thyme

1 Tbsp dried oregano

1 Tbsp dried basil

2 Tbsp dried turmeric

> Sauté onions, green onions, and garlic in pan on low heat for 10 minutes.
> Add in eggs, cheese, and herbs.
> Cook for 10 minutes and add in turmeric.
> Serves 1.

Sage Chicken Breakfast Patties

1 lb of pasture-raised ground chicken, light and dark meat

¼ tsp freshly ground pepper

¼ tsp sea salt

1 tsp ground sage

½ tsp onion powder

¼ tsp garlic powder

¼ tsp dried basil

1 Tbsp fresh Italian parsley

1 large apple, peeled and diced

> Combine all the ingredients in bowl and mix with hands. Shape into patties the size of breakfast sausage patties.
> Heat a large skillet on medium-high heat with coconut oil. Add your chicken patties and cook for approximately 6-8 minutes on each side.
> Serves 4.

BAKED APPLE CINNAMON OATMEAL

PEANUT BUTTER SYRUP

Baked Apple Cinnamon Oatmeal

4 cups Amasai or sheep milk yogurt

½ cup coconut sugar

2 Tbsp grass-fed butter

¾ tsp cinnamon

¼ tsp nutmeg

⅛ tsp cardamom

2 cups old fashioned oats

2 cups chopped apples

½ cup raisins

1 cup chopped nuts

½ tsp sea salt

> Preheat oven to 350. Bring Amasai, coconut sugar, butter, salt, nutmeg, cardamom, and cinnamon to a boil in pot. Add remaining ingredients and bake in buttered casserole dish for 30-35 minutes.

> Serves 4-5.

Peanut Butter Syrup

1 cup organic maple syrup or 1 cup raw, unheated honey

¼ cup raw peanut butter

1 Tbsp butter

1 tsp vanilla

> In medium saucepan over medium-high heat, whisk together all ingredients except vanilla, and bring to a boil.

> Boil 1 minute.

> Add vanilla.

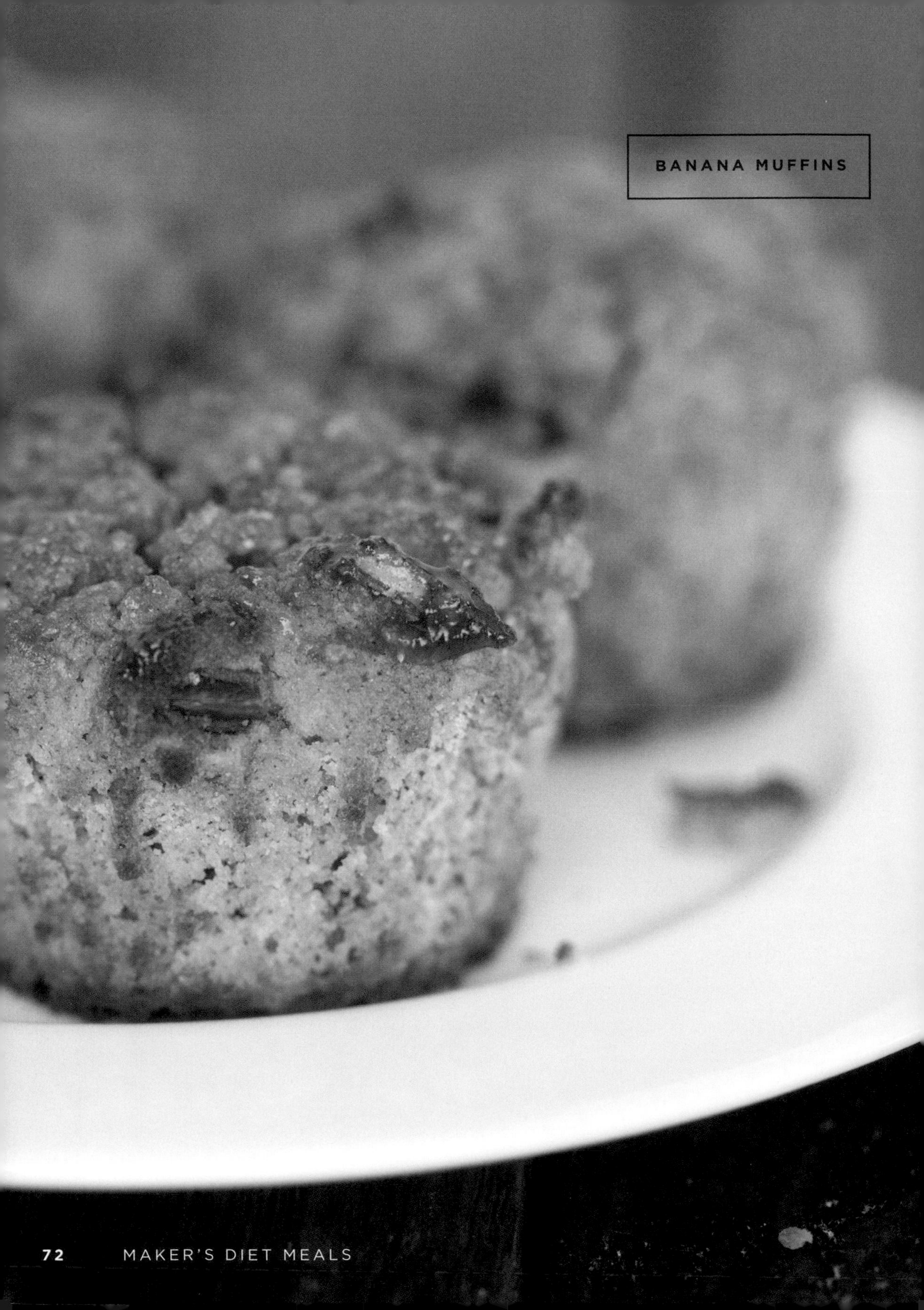
BANANA MUFFINS

Banana Muffins

½ cup grass-fed butter, softened

½ cup coconut sugar

1 tsp vanilla extract

3 pastured eggs, well beaten

¾ cup sprouted omega flour (see recipe on page 204) or coconut flour

1 tsp baking soda

½ tsp sea salt

3 ripe bananas

½ cup walnuts, roughly chopped

> In mixer bowl, beat together butter and coconut sugar until well combined and fluffy. Cut each banana into about 3-4 pieces and add to butter/coconut sugar mixture. Beat until well combined. Add vanilla and eggs and continue to mix.

> In separate small bowl, add coconut flour with baking soda and salt. Mix the flour mixture by hand into the egg/coconut sugar mixture. Stir walnuts into the dough.

> Lightly oil paper muffin cups with coconut oil. Fill muffin cups to the top of paper. Bake at 350 for 20-25 minutes.

> Makes 12 muffins.

Superfood Muffins

4 pastured eggs

⅔ cup coconut oil

1 Tbsp vanilla extract

⅓ cup coconut flour

½ cup gogi berries (dried)

½ cup blueberries

½ cup coconut sugar

1 tsp sea salt

1 tsp baking powder

2 drops orange essential oil

> Whisk eggs, melted coconut oil, vanilla, orange oil, and coconut sugar in a bowl.

> Add in coconut flour and whisk well.

> Let it thicken for 5 minutes.

> Add in the berries and baking powder.

> Line a muffin tin with muffin cups.

> Spoon batter into the muffin cups and bake at 350 for 10 minutes.

> Serves 4.

FRUIT PARFAIT

BANANA NUT BREAD

Fruit Parfait

1 cup berries

½ cup raw pecans

1 cup Amasai or sheep milk yogurt

1 Tbsp raw, unheated honey

> Place nuts and berries in bowl.
> Pour Amasai over the top.

Banana Nut Bread

6 pastured eggs

1 ½ cups melted ghee/butter

2 really ripe bananas

1 Tbsp vanilla extract

½ tsp Himilayan salt

1 cup blanched almond flour

½ cup coconut flour

1 tsp baking powder

½ cup walnuts

1 cup organic dark chocolate chips

> In a high-speed blender, blend eggs, melted butter/ghee, bananas, and vanilla together.
> Pour mixture into a bowl and whisk in flours and baking powder.
> Let it sit for 10 minutes to thicken.
> Add in chocolate chips and nuts.
> Pour into a greased loaf pan and bake for 20 minutes at 350 degrees.
> Serves 4.

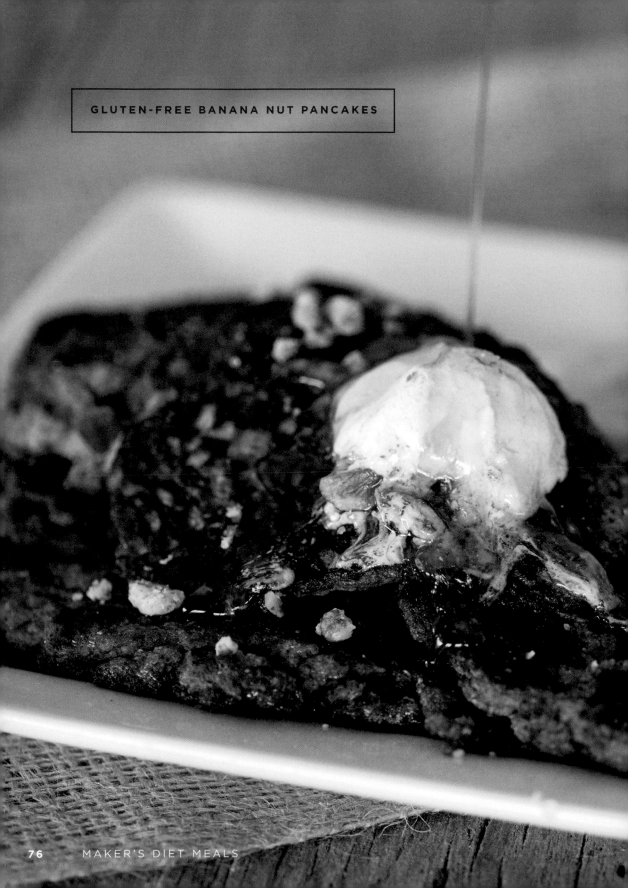

GLUTEN-FREE BANANA NUT PANCAKES

Gluten-Free Banana Nut Pancakes

½ cup cooked quinoa

2 ripe bananas, mashed

2 Tbsp coconut oil, melted

2 Tbsp coconut sugar

1 Tbsp lemon juice

2 pastured eggs, well beaten

1 cup oat flour, sprouted omega flour (page 204), or coconut flour

½ tsp baking soda

½ tsp fine sea salt

½ tsp ground cinnamon

¼ tsp nutmeg

½ cup Amasai or coconut milk

½ rough chopped walnuts

PEANUT BUTTER SYRUP:

1 cup maple syrup or raw, unheated honey

¼ cup peanut butter

1 Tbsp grass-fed butter

1 tsp vanilla extract

CINNAMON SYRUP:

1 cup maple syrup or raw, unheated honey

1 tsp cinnamon

¼ tsp nutmeg

1 Tbsp grass-fed butter

1 tsp vanilla extract

> Put all ingredients in large bowl. Stir gently but thoroughly. Do not over stir or mixture will be tough. Put your griddle on medium heat and add in coconut oil. When griddle is hot, place about ¼ cup of the batter on the griddle.

> Cook pancakes about 3 minutes first side and about 1 minute on other side or until middle is no longer doughy. Serve with peanut butter syrup or cinnamon syrup.

> PEANUT BUTTER SYRUP: In medium saucepan over medium-high heat, whisk together all ingredients except vanilla, and bring to a boil. Boil 1 minute. Add vanilla.

> CINNAMON SYRUP: In medium saucepan, over medium-high heat, whisk all ingredients together except the vanilla. Bring to a boil and boil for one minute. Take off heat and add vanilla.

> Serves 4.

Tomato Basil Omelet

1 small tomato, chopped

1 tsp dried basil

1 tsp fresh garlic

1 tsp sea salt

3 pastured eggs

1 Tbsp coconut oil

> In a frying pan place oil to melt on medium heat.
> Whisk eggs together with basil, garlic, and salt.
> Pour into the pan.
> When nearly cooked, add tomatoes to the middle of the eggs.
> Flip eggs over to form an omelet.
> Serve with green-fed, raw cheddar or goat cheese
> Serves 2.

Grain Free Pumpkin Spice Muffins

⅔ cup canned pumpkin puree

½ cup coconut oil

½ cup raw, unheated honey

1 Tbsp vanilla extract

4 pastured eggs

⅓ cup coconut flour

1 tsp baking powder

1 tsp ginger

1 tsp cinnamon

1 tsp nutmeg

1 tsp sea salt

> Blend pumpkin, oil, honey, vanilla, eggs, salt, and spices in a high-speed mixer until smooth.
> Pour mixture into a large bowl, add flour and baking powder.
> Pour into a muffin pan and bake for 15 minutes at 325 degrees.
> Serve with butter on top.
> Serves 6.

Probiotic Blueberry Muffins

3 pastured eggs

½ cup melted coconut oil

¼ cup cultured whey or Ama-sai

½ cup raw, unheated honey

½ tsp sea salt

½ cup blueberries

½ cup coconut flour

¾ tsp baking powder

> Combine, eggs, coconut oil, cultured whey, honey, and salt together.
> Add flour and baking powder and let it thicken for 5 minutes.
> Add blueberries and bake at 325 for 15-20 minutes.
> Serves 4.

Probiotic Blueberry Pancakes

2 pastured eggs

2 Tbsp Amasai or sheep milk yogurt

2 Tbsp coconut oil

2 Tbsp raw, unheated honey

⅛ tsp sea salt

2 Tbsp coconut flour

⅛ tsp baking powder

¼ cup blueberries

> Mix all wet ingredients together in a large bowl.
> Add flour, salt, baking powder, and berries.
> Pour onto a greased skillet (greased with coconut oil) on low heat.
> Flip and serve!
> Serves 2.

Breakfast Casserole

10 pastured eggs

1 lb. grass-fed ground beef

8 oz Amasai or sheep milk yogurt

6 oz green-fed, raw cheddar cheese or goat cheese shredded (2 cups)

½ tsp sea salt

1 tsp nutmeg

½ tsp black pepper

> Whisk eggs, Amasai, nutmeg, pepper, and salt together.
> Spread the ground beef evenly in a greased baking dish (greased with coconut oil).
> Pour eggs over the beef.
> Sprinkle the cheese evenly on top.
> Bake at 350 for 15-20 minutes.
> Serves 6.

Apple Cinnamon Breakfast Muffins

1 apple, cored

3 dates

1 Tbsp vanilla extract

⅔ cup melted grass-fed butter

4 pastured eggs

½ tsp sea salt

1 Tbsp cinnamon

½ cup coconut flour

1 tsp baking powder

> In a blender, place apple, dates, vanilla, melted butter, eggs, and salt.
> Blend well.
> Pour into a bowl and whisk in flour.
> Let it thicken for 5 minutes.
> Add cinnamon and baking powder.
> Spoon into greased muffin tin and bake at 350 for 10 minutes.
> Makes 8-12 muffins.

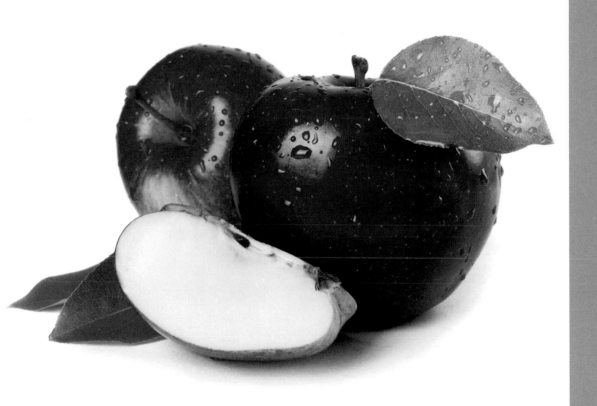

desserts

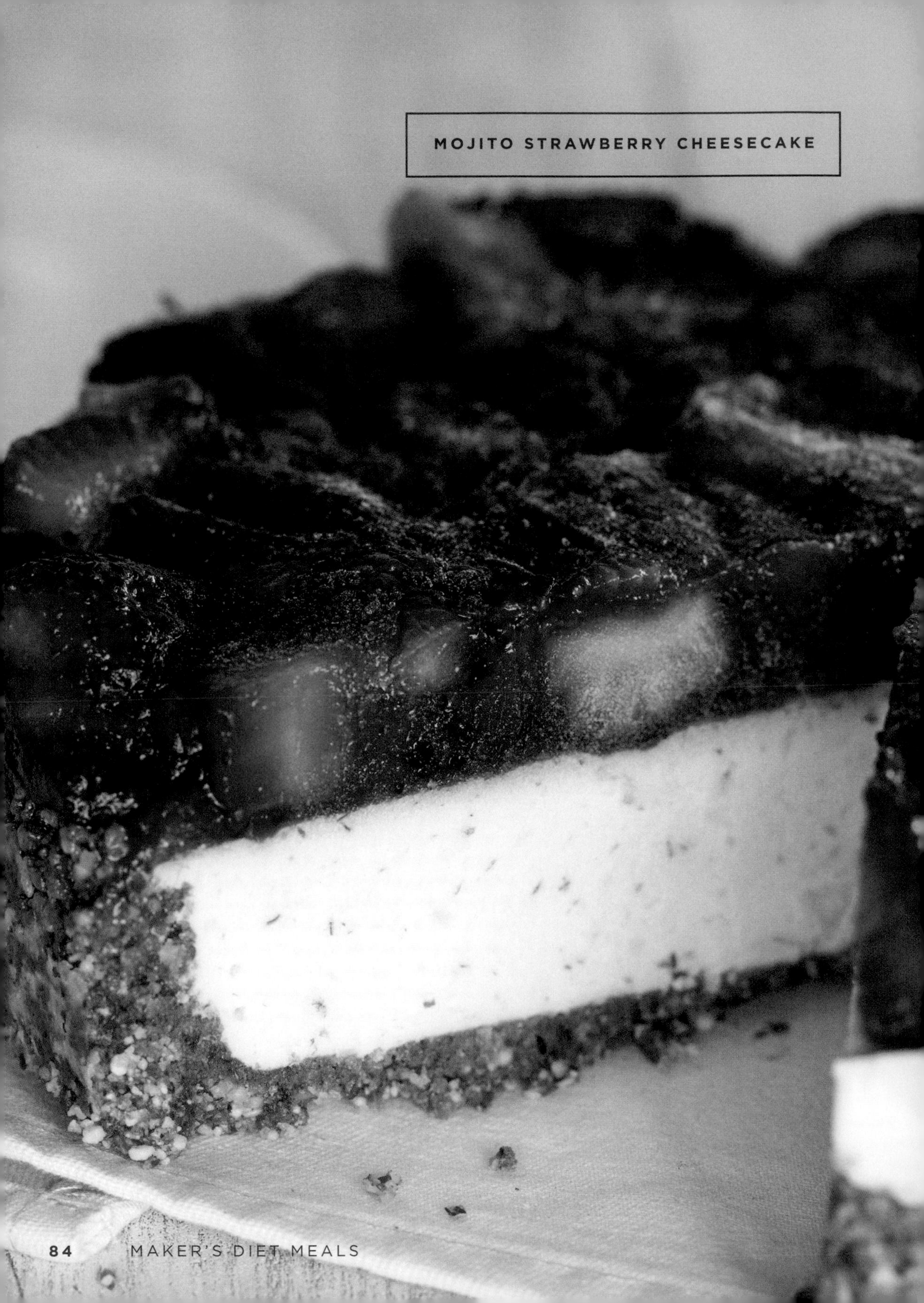

Mojito Strawberry Cheesecake

CRUST:

2 cups almonds

1 cup dates, pits removed

1 tsp vanilla extract

1 Tbsp raw, unheated honey

MOJITO LIME FILLING:

6 Tbsp unsalted grass-fed butter, softened

¾ cup coconut sugar

½ cup raw, unheated honey

2 pastured eggs

6 pastured egg yolks

1 cup fresh squeezed lime juice

2 Tbsp tapioca starch

½ cup coconut heavy cream (the cream on top of the can of coconut milk)

⅓ cup coconut oil

STRAWBERRY GLAZE:

1 10-oz package frozen whole strawberries

16 oz fresh strawberries

1 tsp fresh squeezed lime juice

¼ cup coconut sugar or raw, unheated honey

1 Tbsp tapioca starch

2 Tbsp fresh mint, finely chopped

> CRUST: Put all ingredients in food processor and blend until sticky. Lightly oil a nine-inch cheesecake pan with coconut oil. Press the crust dough into the cheesecake pan. Place dough in freezer while you make the filling.

> MOJITO LIME FILLING: In mixing bowl, beat the butter, coconut sugar, and honey with electric mixer for about 2 minutes or until well blended and mixed. Add eggs and yolks to the butter mixture and beat until well blended.

> In separate bowl, add tapioca starch to the lime juice, stir well until tapioca starch is dissolved. Add the lime juice mixture to the butter mixture and continue to beat for about 1 minute.

> Pour the mixture into a medium heavy saucepan and cook over low-medium heat, stirring constantly, until mixture thickens and looks smooth. When done, remove pan from stove to cool. Fold in coconut cream and coconut oil until totally blended.

> Remove the crust from the freezer and put the filling into the crust. Return cheesecake to freezer and let freeze for about 5-6 hours or overnight.

(cont.)

Raw Mojito Strawberry Cheesecake (cont.)

> Thaw frozen strawberries in a fine strainer over bowl. When thawed, press strawberries through the strainer into the juice below until you get ½ cup of strawberry juice. Set strawberries that remain in strainer aside. You will use them later.

> To the ½ cup juice add tapioca starch. Pour the mixture into a small saucepan on medium heat and bring to a boil, stirring occasionally. Reduce heat and simmer for approximately 4 minutes stirring occasionally until mixture is thickened.

> Slice the fresh strawberries and gently mix them together with the remaining pulp saved in the strainer. Add ¼ cup coconut sugar (or raw, unheated honey) and stir gently to coat the strawberries. Let stand for about 10 minutes so sugar will dissolve. Add lime juice and finely minced mint and stir. Add the cooled strawberry mixture. Spread strawberry mixture over entire lime cheesecake top. Return to freezer for at least 2 hours.

> Serves 8.

Frozen Fruit

1 bag of grapes

1 mango

1 watermelon

> Wash grapes and freeze on baking tray.

> Peel one mango. Cut the fruit away from the seed and cut into long strips. Place on baking sheet and freeze.

> Cut rind off of watermelon and cut into large pieces about two inches each. Place on baking sheet and freeze.

> When completely frozen, place in bags and store in freezer.

Raw Pumpkin Cheesecake

CRUST:

2 cups pecans

15 medjool dates, pitted

1 Tbsp raw, unheated honey

4 Tbsp hemp seeds

½ tsp ginger

¼ tsp nutmeg

1 tsp cinnamon

1 tsp vanilla extract

PUMPKIN FILLING:

1 ½ cups cashews, soaked for at least 8 hours

½ cup raw, unheated honey

1 ¼ cup canned pumpkin

¼ cup coconut oil

1 ½ tsp cinnamon

¼ tsp ginger

⅛ tsp cloves

¼ tsp sea salt

2 tsp vanilla extract

½ cup coconut cream (the cream on top of the can of coconut milk)

> CRUST: Grind nuts in food processor and add the rest of the ingredients. Process until the mixture begins to stick. Pack the date mixture tightly on bottom and about one inch up the sides of the pan. Put in freezer until filling is ready.

> PUMPKIN FILLING: Thoroughly rinse and drain cashews. Blend in a food processor until cashews are finely ground up. Add the coconut cream and process until cashews are creamy.

> Add remaining ingredients and process until mixture is creamy. Pour pumpkin filling into well chilled pie crust. Freeze for at least 3 hours.

> Serves about 8.

CHOCOLATE COCONUT COOKIES

STRAWBERRY MILK SHAKE

Chocolate Coconut Cookies

½ cup ghee/coconut oil, melted

¾ cup coconut sugar

4 pastured eggs

½ tsp vanilla

½ cup coconut flour

2 cups organic unsweetened coconut flakes

1 cup organic dark chocolate chips

> Mix eggs, coconut sugar, melted oil/ghee, and vanilla together in a mixer.
> Add coconut flour and flakes. Mix well.
> Drop by spoonfuls on a pan and form into cookies.
> Bake at 375 degrees for 15-20 minutes.
> Melt chocolate chips over the stove and drizzle over cookie.
> Serves 4.

Strawberry Milk Shake

1 cup strawberries

½ banana

1 cup Amasai or coconut cream (the cream on top of the can of coconut milk)

1 cup ice

1 tsp vanilla

> Blend in blender.

STRAWBERRY SHORTCAKE CUPCAKES

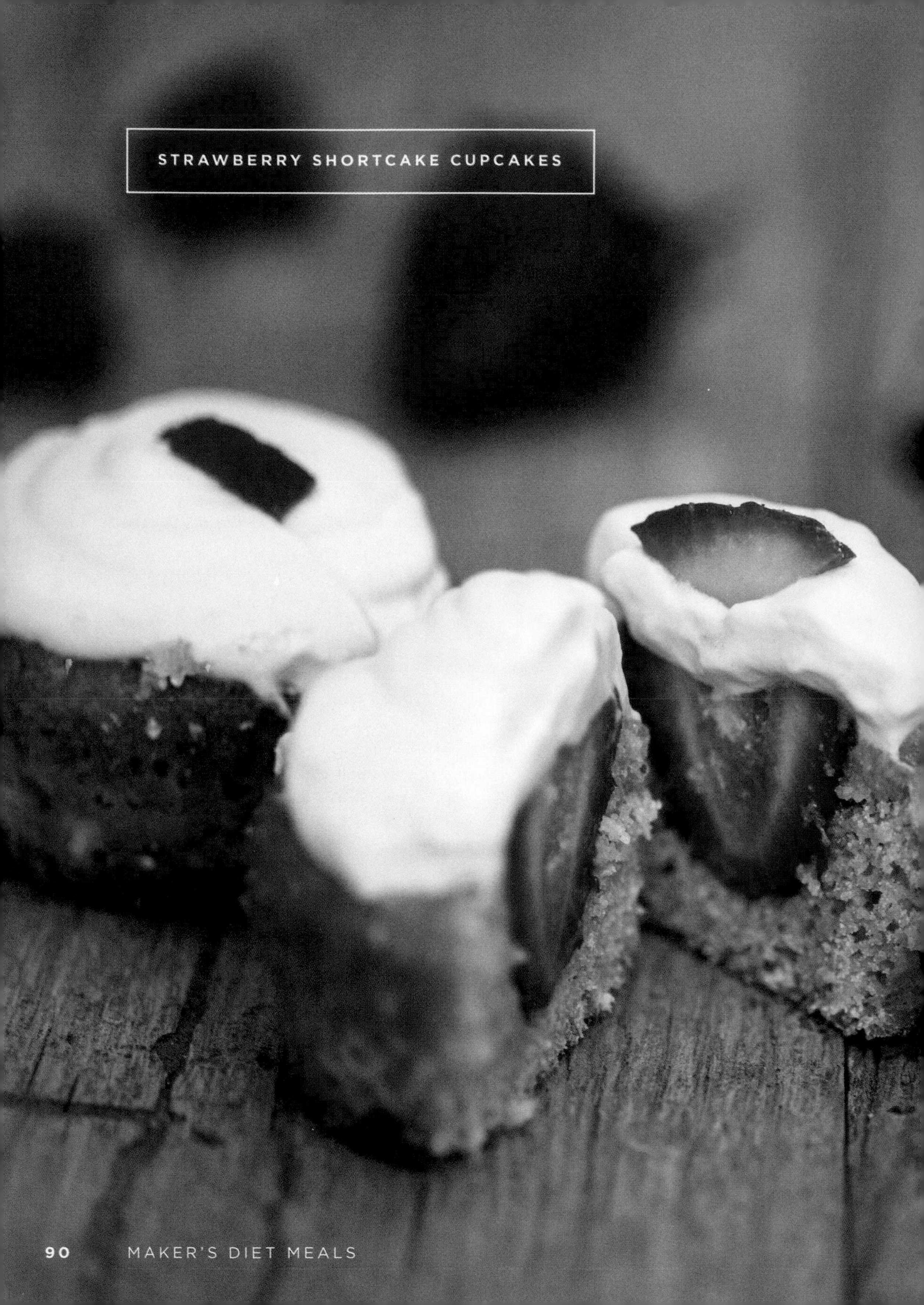

Strawberry Shortcake Cupcakes

½ cup sprouted omega flour
(page 204) or coconut flour

¼ tsp baking soda

¼ tsp sea salt

5 pastured eggs

½ cup raw, unheated honey

½ cup coconut oil

¼ cup flaked organic coconut

1 tsp lemon juice

1 tsp vanilla extract

12 whole strawberries

2 cups whipped coconut
cream (the cream on top of
the can of coconut milk)

> Preheat your oven to 350 degrees.

> Place 12 cupcake liners in a muffin pan.

> Sift dry ingredients together into a
  bowl. Add the coconut separately.

> Separate 2 of the eggs. Set the egg
  whites aside.

> Combine 3 eggs, two egg yolks,
  coconut oil, honey, vanilla, and lemon
  juice with a hand mixer. Be careful that
  you don't over mix.

> Turn the mixer to low and add the dry
  mixture and wet mixture in alternate
  batches until the batter has no lumps.

> In a small bowl beat the egg whites
  until thick, soft peaks form. (Using a
  hand mixer works best.) Fold into the
  batter very gently.

> Pour or spoon batter evenly into the 12
  cupcake liners.

> Bake at 350 degrees for about 20
  minutes. Check if your cupcakes are
  done by putting a toothpick in the
  center of one. If it comes out clean, the
  cupcakes are finished. Allow to cool
  for 5-10 minutes, then carefully remove
  cupcakes from the pan. Let cool
  completely.

> When the cupcakes are cool, cut a
  small circle off the top and scoop out
  a little of the cupcake to fit one whole
  strawberry.

> Use your whipped coconut cream as a
  frosting. When you cut the cupcake in
  half, you see the pretty red strawberry.
  It looks like a miniature strawberry
  shortcake!

> You can chill the cupcakes before you
  put the strawberries in and frost them.

> Makes approximately 12 cupcakes.

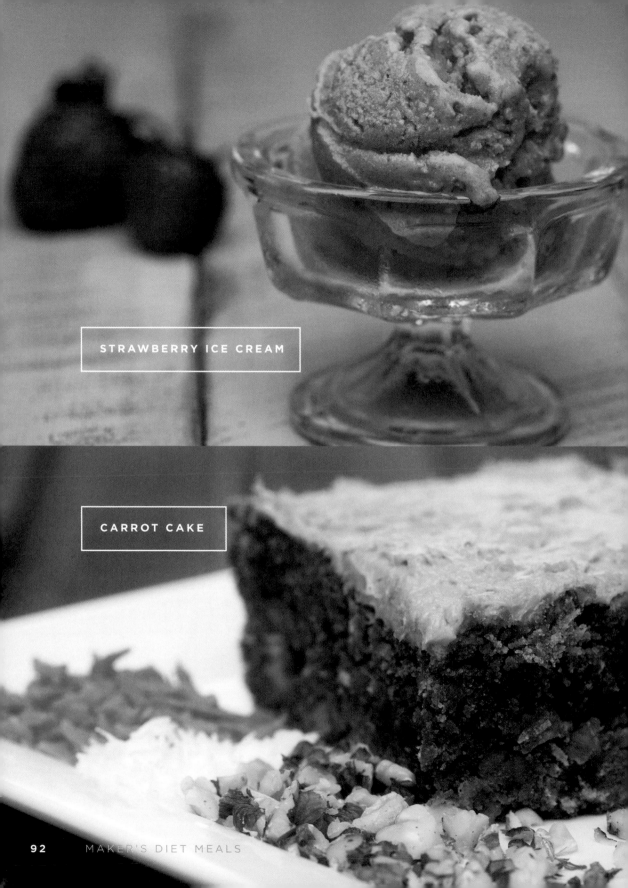

STRAWBERRY ICE CREAM

CARROT CAKE

Strawberry Ice Cream

½ cup raw, unheated honey

½ cup fresh squeezed orange juice

16 oz plain Amasai or sheep milk yogurt

½ ripe banana, frozen

4 cups strawberries, frozen

> Put all ingredients in food processor or blender and blend. Pour mixture into a medium-sized glass baking dish, cover, and put in freezer. Take out about 10 minutes before you plan to serve it and blend again.

> Serves 4.

Carrot Cake

3 cups whole spelt flour or whole wheat pastry flour

2 ¼ cups coconut sugar

1 tsp sea salt

1 Tbsp baking soda

1 Tbsp cinnamon

1 ½ cups coconut oil

4 pastured eggs, lightly beaten

1 Tbsp vanilla extract

1 ½ cups chopped raw or sprouted walnuts or pecans

1 ½ cups shredded coconut

1 ⅓ cups shredded raw carrots

¾ cup crushed pineapple

TIPS:
- You can use walnuts or pecans.
- If you like raisins, feel free to add them as well.
- If you don't like pineapple, try ripe banana.
- This cake freezes exceptionally well. Cut into individual squares, wrap each one, and freeze in a gallon ziplock bag.
- You can also use this recipe for cupcakes. It makes 24. Bake about 25-30 minutes.

> Preheat oven to 350. Grease two nine-inch layer cake pans and line with waxed paper or grease a large 9 x 13 inch pyrex or sheet pan. No need to use waxed paper if you're using the large pyrex.

> Sift dry ingredients into a bowl. Add oil, eggs, and vanilla. Beat well. Fold in walnuts, coconut, carrots, and pineapple.

> Pour batter into the prepared pan or pans. Bake for 30-35 minutes or until edges have pulled away from the sides and a cake tester inserted into the middle comes out clean. If you use the 9 x 13 pyrex or the sheet pan cook for 50-60 minutes.

> Cool on a rack for 3 hours. Fill and frost with coconut cream cheese frosting (see recipe on page 82).

> Makes 12-18 good-sized squares.

CINNAMON BUNS WITH CREAM CHEESE FROSTING

Cinnamon Buns with Cream Cheese Frosting

1 cup almond flour

2 Tbsp coconut flour

½ tsp baking soda

¼ tsp sea salt

¼ cup coconut oil

¼ cup coconut sugar

3 pastured eggs

1 Tbsp vanilla extract

> Combine dry ingredients in a large bowl.

> Combine wet ingredients in separate mixing bowl.

> Fold wet ingredients into the dry ingredients and mix well.

> Scoop batter into muffin pan and top with cinnamon topping.

CINNAMON TOPPING:

2 Tbsp maple syrup

1 Tbsp melted ghee

1 Tbsp ground cinnamon

> CINNAMON TOPPING: Mix together and pour over muffins.

> Bake at 350 for 8-12 minutes

> Top with cream cheese frosting

CREAM CHEESE FROSTING:

1 cup strained Amasai or sheep milk yogurt

⅔ cup softened ghee

1 tsp pure vanilla extract

¼ cup coconut sugar

> CREAM CHEESE FROSTING: Mix ingredients together.

> Serves 6.

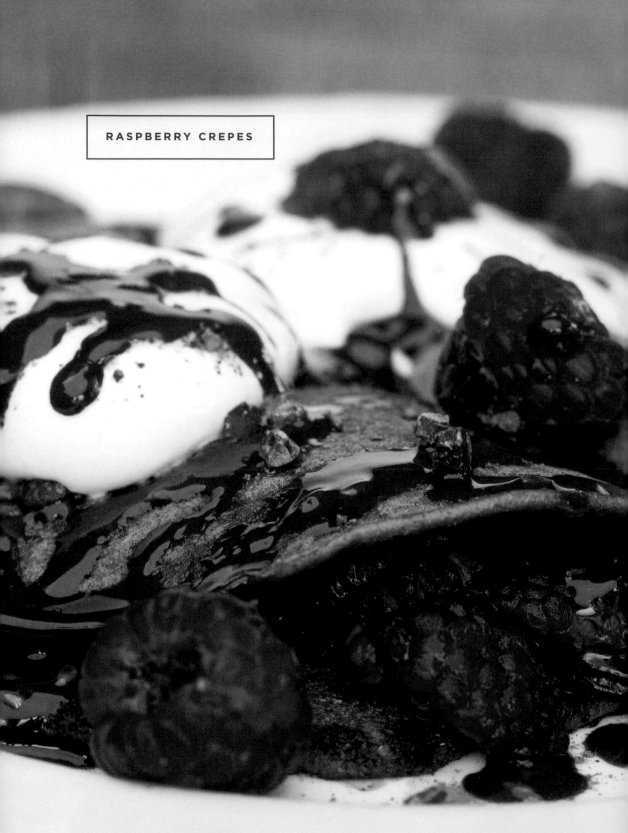

RASPBERRY CREPES

Raspberry Crepes

CREPES:

½ cup cooked quinoa

2 Tbsp coconut oil

1 Tbsp cocoa powder

4 Tbsp raw, unheated honey or maple syrup

2 pastured eggs, well beaten

1 cup oat flour

½ tsp sea salt

½ tsp ground cinnamon

½ tsp vanilla

½ cup Amasai or coconut milk

⅓ cup water

WHIPPED COCONUT CREAM:

1 cup coconut cream

1 tsp vanilla extract

2 Tbsp maple syrup

CHOCOLATE SAUCE:

½ cup raw, unheated honey

½ cup raw cacao powder

2 Tbsp coconut oil, melted

1 tsp vanilla extract

> In medium bowl, mix all ingredients together. Batter should be very thin. Heat small 7-9 inch skillet with coconut oil. When skillet is warm, pour ⅓ cup of batter in skillet. Carefully flip the crepe and cook other side until the consistency is no longer wet.

> WHIPPED COCONUT CREAM: Put a can of coconut milk in the refrigerator for several hours or overnight. Open can and skim off the thick white cream to measure one cup. Mix in mixing bowl with an electric mixer add coconut cream, vanilla, and maple syrup. Whip until cream is soft peaks. Use in many recipes and as a substitute for whipped dairy cream.

> CHOCOLATE SAUCE: In food processor, blend all ingredients together.

> ASSEMBLE: Put one crepe on a dessert plate, fill with a few crushed raspberries, add coconut whipped cream, and fold crepe over in half. Add a dollop of whipped coconut cream and drizzle with chocolate sauce.

> Serves 6.

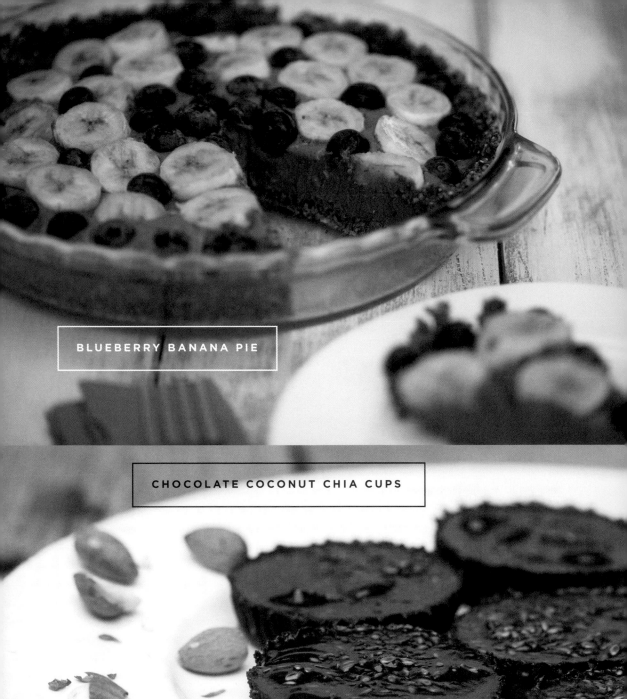

BLUEBERRY BANANA PIE

CHOCOLATE COCONUT CHIA CUPS

Blueberry Banana Pie

PIE CRUST

2 cups ground pecans

½ cup Terrain Omega

6 pitted dates

⅓ cup coconut oil

PIE:

1 cup strained Amasai

⅓ cup coconut sugar

2 peeled bananas

1 cup defrosted frozen blueberries

1 cup heavy coconut cream

⅓ cup raw cane sugar

> PIE CRUST: Blend all ingredients together in food processor until well combined. Spread into pie pan and freeze.

> PIE: In a medium bowl, combine strained Amasai and ⅓ cup coconut sugar. Beat until fluffy. Spoon mixture into raw pie shell and spread evenly. Arrange banana slices on cream cheese layer. Spread blueberries on top of banana slices.

> In a medium bowl, combine whipping cream and ⅓ cup raw cane sugar. Beat until stiff. Spread whipped cream on top of pie. Chill in refrigerator until ready to serve.

Chocolate Coconut Chia Cups

1 cup coconut butter

½ cup coconut oil

½ cup raw cacao powder

⅔ cup Terrain Omega or ground chia seeds

1 Tbsp raw, unheated honey

Dash sea salt

> Mix all ingredients together!
> Spoon into candy molds and freeze for 10 minutes.
> If you don't have candy molds, just roll them into balls!
> TIP: You might have to warm the coconut butter under warm water to melt it a bit.

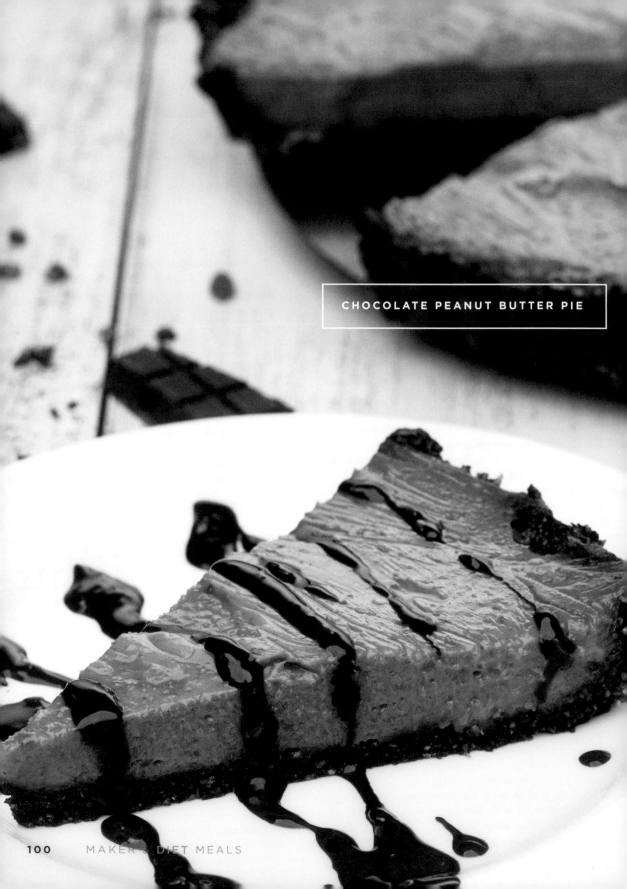

CHOCOLATE PEANUT BUTTER PIE

Chocolate Peanut Butter Pie

CRUST:

10-12 medjool dates, pitted

1 cup ground walnuts

1 cup ground pecans

2 Tbsp hemp seeds

¼ cup raw cacao powder

¼ cup raw, unheated honey

1 tsp vanilla extract

PEANUT BUTTER FILLING:

1 cup peanut butter

3 ripe bananas

1 ½ tsp vanilla extract

¼ cup coconut oil, melted

¼ cup raw, unheated honey

CHOCOLATE GLAZE:

1 cup raw, unheated honey

1 cup raw cacao powder

¼ cup coconut oil, melted

1 Tbsp vanilla extract

> CRUST: Put walnuts and pecans in food processor and blend. Add rest of ingredients to food processor and process until mixture is sticky. Do not over process. Grease a nine-inch springform pan with coconut oil. Firmly pat dough into pan and up the sides about an inch. Place pan into freezer while making the filling.

> PEANUT BUTTER FILLING: Blend all filling ingredients in food processor or blender until well combined and creamy. Pour filling into the chocolate crust. Place pie in freezer.

> CHOCOLATE GLAZE: In food processor, blend all ingredients together. Spoon over peanut butter pie.

> Serves 8-10

Apple/Cherry Crisp

4 cups tart apples, peeled and sliced

2 cups frozen cherries, thawed

Juice of 1 lemon

1 Tbsp cinnamon

½ tsp nutmeg

⅛ tsp ginger

½ tsp sea salt

2 Tbsp tapioca starch

½ cup frozen apple juice concentrate, thawed

TOPPING:

1 cup rolled oats

4 Tbsp hemp seeds

2 Tbsp coconut flour

½ cup walnuts, chopped

⅓ cup coconut sugar

1 tsp cinnamon

¼ cup grass-fed butter, melted

> Toss all ingredients together. Spread in a lightly greased nine-inch glass baking dish. Bake in oven at 375 for 30 minutes. Take out of oven and add topping to the top of the hot fruit. Return to oven and bake for 15 minutes more, until topping is browned.

> TOPPING: Mix all ingredients together, except melted butter. Mix well. Add melted butter and mix again until it is crumbly and blended together.

> Serves 6-8.

Peppermint Squares

1 cup coconut oil

2 drops peppermint essential oil

1 Tbsp raw, unheated honey

Pinch of sea salt

2 bars of dark chocolate

> Mix all ingredients (minus chocolate) in a bowl.

> Melt 2 dark chocolate bars with 1 Tbsp coconut oil.

> Spoon into candy mold and freeze.

> Spoon peppermint mixture on top and freeze.

> Serves 8.

Blackberry Banana Ice Cream

½ cup raw, unheated honey or coconut sugar

2 cups fresh squeezed orange juice

4 cups Amasai or coconut milk

2 ripe bananas, frozen

¾ cup blackberries, frozen

> In a blender, blend all ingredients together until creamy. Pour into a glass container and cover. Freeze for at least 4 hours or overnight. Just before serving, you may re-blend mixture to make it creamier.

> Serves 4.

Cherry Ice Cream

2 cups black cherries, frozen

½ cup freshly squeezed orange juice

½ ripe banana, frozen

⅓ cup raw, unheated honey or coconut sugar

1 ½ cups Amasai or coconut milk

> Put all ingredients in blender and blend until smooth. Place in glass bowl and cover. Freeze until serving time. Place back in blender or food processor and process until creamy just before serving.

> Serves 6.

Mango Peach Ice Cream

5 ripe mangoes

16 oz Amasai, coconut milk, or sheep milk yogurt

2 Tbsp fresh squeezed lime juice

1 cup peaches, drained

¼ cup raw, unheated honey

¼ cup coconut sugar

½ cup water

1 ripe banana

> Blend all ingredients in food processor until creamy.

> Freeze the mixture in a shallow metal pan until frozen. Right before serving, break ice cream up into chunks and process in food processor until smooth.

> Serves 4.

Chia Pudding with Fruit

1 ½ cups coconut milk

3 Tbsp chia seeds

4 dried apricots, pitted

3 dates, pitted

1 Tbsp maple syrup

¼ tsp sea salt

½ tsp cinnamon

¼ tsp nutmeg

3 Tbsp walnuts, rough chopped, soaked, and dehydrated or toasted

½ cup fresh cherries, pitted and cut in half

¼ cup fresh mango, diced

> In a blender, place the coconut milk, chia seeds, apricots, dates, maple syrup, sea salt, cinnamon, and nutmeg and blend on high speed until smooth.

> Put mixture in small bowl, cover, and let sit in refrigerator for at least 8 hours. Right before serving, add the chopped walnuts, cherries, and mangos. Serve cold.

> Serves 2-3.

High Fiber Raw Chocolate Fudge

1 cup coconut butter

½ cup coconut oil

½ cup raw cacao powder

⅔ cup ground chia seeds

1 Tbsp raw, unheated honey

Dash sea salt

> Mix all ingredients together.

> Spoon into candy molds and freeze for 10 minutes.

> If you don't have candy molds, just roll them into balls!

> TIP: You might have to warm the coconut butter under warm water to melt it a bit.

> Serves 8.

Lemon Passion Tea Tart

CRUST:

2 cups almonds

1 cup medjool dates, pits removed

1 tsp vanilla extract

1 Tbsp raw, unheated honey

LEMON PASSION FRUIT FILLING:

2 cups of raw cashews, soaked in purified water for at least 4-8 hours.

5 passion fruit tea bags

1 cup purified water

2 Tbsp lemon zest

1 tsp vanilla extract

⅓ cup fresh squeezed lemon juice

⅓ cup raw, unheated honey

½ cup coconut oil

¼ tsp sea salt

> Place almonds in the food processor until nuts are finely chopped. Add the rest of the ingredients and process until the mixture is sticky. Lightly grease a tart pan with coconut oil and press crust mixture into pan. Refrigerate for about an hour to help set it.

> FRUIT FILLING: Thoroughly rinse the cashews and drain. Set aside.

> Bring 1 cup filtered water to a boil in small saucepan. When water comes to boil, turn off heat and submerge the tea bags. Let steep for at least 10 minutes or until they cool down.

> Squeeze the water out of the tea bags. Carefully open tea bags and empty contents into the steeped tea.

> Put the drained cashews in food processor and process until cashews are creamy and smooth. Add the tea, lemon juice, vanilla, raw, unheated honey, coconut oil, and salt and process until very creamy. Add the lemon zest and pulse once or twice until it is incorporated in the filling.

> Fill the crust with passion fruit filling. Top with one cup heavy coconut cream, ½ tsp lemon extract, 2 Tbsp lemon zest, 4 Tbsp fresh lemon juice, and ¼ cup raw, unheated honey. Whip and garnish with lemon zest.

> Serves 8.

Peanut Butter Brownie

15 oz chickpeas, rinsed and drained

½ cup peanut butter

¼ cup coconut sugar

⅓ cup raw, unheated honey

2 Tbsp raw cacao powder

1 Tbsp vanilla extract

¼ tsp baking soda

¼ tsp non-aluminum baking powder

½ cup soaked and dehydrated or toasted walnuts, rough chopped

¼ cup cacao nibs or dark chocolate pieces

PEANUT BUTTER GLAZE:

¼ cup maple syrup

¼ cup peanut butter

> In a food processor, blend chickpeas until smooth. Add all ingredients except cacao nibs and toasted walnuts. Process until smooth.

> Place dough in a medium-sized bowl and stir in cacao nibs and toasted walnuts.

> Spread batter in pan coated in coconut oil. Bake at 350 for 25-28 minutes.

> PEANUT BUTTER GLAZE: Place both ingredients in small bowl, stirring constantly until thoroughly mixed. Lightly brush glaze on cooled bars.

> Makes approximately 14 bars

Peanut Butter Cookie

2 cups peanut butter

1 cup raw, unheated honey

2 pastured eggs, beaten

⅛ cup coconut flour

2 tsp baking soda

1 tsp vanilla extract

> In a small bowl, whisk the flour and baking soda together.

> In separate bowl, mix all other ingredients together. Add the flour to the peanut butter mixture and stir well.

> Bake at 350 for 8 minutes.

> Makes approximately 12 cookies.

Peanut Butter Ball Bites

½ cup old fashioned oats

½ cup freshly ground peanut butter

¼ cup flax or chia meal

2 Tbsp raw, unheated honey

3 Tbsp hemp seeds

2 Tbsp raw cacao powder

1 Tbsp coconut flakes

2 Tbsp coconut oil

1 tsp vanilla extract

> Mix all your ingredients together, except the coconut flakes, until combined thoroughly. Put mixture in the refrigerator for 1 hour.

> Roll into medium-sized balls the size of a walnut and refrigerate until set. Store in an airtight container in the refrigerator.

> Makes 12-14 balls.

Grandma's Chocolate Raisin Cake

8 pastured eggs

½ cup melted coconut oil

½ cup plain Amasai or sheep milk yogurt

½ cup coconut nectar or maple syrup

1 Tbsp vanilla extract

2 cups almond flour

½ cup raw cacao powder

¼ cup coconut sugar

½ cup raisins

⅔ cup raw walnuts

⅔ cup 70% dark chocolate chips

1 tsp baking powder

1 tsp sea salt

> Mix together almond flour, raisins, cacao powder, coconut sugar, walnuts, chocolate chips, baking powder, and salt.

> In a separate bowl, whisk eggs, melted oil, Amasai, coconut nectar or maple syrup, and vanilla extract.

> Combine dry ingredients.

> Mix together well.

> In a greased cake pan (greased with coconut oil), pour in batter.

> Bake at 350 for 20-30 minutes.

> Serves 6.

Vanilla Cupcakes

6 pastured eggs

1 cup almond flour

½ cup coconut flour

1 Tbsp vanilla extract

3 Tbsp raw, unheated honey

½ cup plain Amasai or sheep milk yogurt

1 tsp baking powder (aluminum free)

1 tsp sea salt

> Whisk eggs, honey, Amasai, and vanilla together.
> Add in flours, baking powder, and salt.
> Let it sit for 10 minutes.
> Spoon into muffin tin and bake at 350 for 15 minutes.
> Let cool and top with raw chocolate frosting.
> Serves 8.

Brain Boosting Blueberry Pudding

1 cup coconut milk

1 cup plain Amasai or sheep milk yogurt

3 avocados

1 cup blueberries

4 Tbsp ground chia seeds

½ tsp sea salt

1 Tbsp of vanilla extract

1 Tbsp Terrain Fermented Peppermint (optional)

1 tbsp raw, unheated honey or coconut sugar

> Blend all ingredients together in a high powered blender.
> Refrigerate for 12 hours.
> Serves 6.

Birthday Cake

5 pastured eggs

1 cup melted coconut oil

½ cup raw, unheated honey

1 Tbsp vanilla extract

½ tsp sea salt

½ cup coconut flour

1 tsp baking powder

BUTTERCREAM FROSTING:

½ cup softened coconut butter (not oil)

⅔ cup softened grass-fed butter

1 tsp vanilla extract

4 Tbsp raw, unheated honey

¼ cup arrowroot powder

CHOCOLATE TOPPING:

1 bar of dark chocolate

1 tsp coconut oil

> Whisk eggs, oil, honey, vanilla, and salt together.

> Mix in flour and baking powder and mix well.

> Let it sit for 5-10 minutes until thickened.

> Pour into greased mini cake pan and bake for 15 to 20 minutes at 350 degrees.

> BUTTERCREAM FROSTING: In an electric mixer, combine softened butter, softened coconut butter, vanilla, and honey.

> Add in arrowroot powder and mix until smooth.

> Spread over cake after it has been COOLED!

> Refrigerate for 1 hour.

> CHOCOLATE TOPPING: Melt one bar of dark chocolate with 1 tsp coconut oil.

> Pour over refrigerated cake and place in the freezer for 20 minutes.

> Serves 6.

Raw Chocolate Frosting

2 avocados

14 oz coconut milk

1 Tbsp vanilla extract

½ cup raw cacao powder

4 pitted dates

½ tsp sea salt

> Blend in a high-speed blender.

Orange Cake with Butter Cream Frosting

4 pastured eggs

¾ cup clarified butter (ghee)

¼ cup raw, unheated honey

½ tsp sea salt

8 drops orange essential oil

½ cup coconut flour

1 tsp baking powder

BUTTERCREAM FROSTING:

½ cup grass-fed butter (soft, not melted)

1 cup softened coconut milk (canned, full fat)

¼ cup arrowroot powder

1 Tbsp vanilla extract

3 Tbsp coconut sugar

> Whisk eggs, melted oil/butter, honey, salt, and orange oil.
> Add coconut flour and baking powder and whisk well.
> Let it thicken for 5 minutes.
> Pour into a mini cake pan (greased with coconut oil).
> Bake at 350 for 20 minutes.
> Top with buttercream frosting.
> BUTTERCREAM FROSTING: In a mixer, mix butter, coconut cream, arrowroot powder, vanilla, and coconut sugar.
> Spread over cake.
> Variations: Add lemon essential oil and make it a lemon cake.
> Serves 8.

Brownies

5 pastured eggs

½ cup melted grass-fed butter or coconut oil

1 Tbsp vanilla extract

⅔ cup coconut sugar

½ cup raw cacao powder

½ cup coconut flour

½ tsp sea salt

¾ cup dark chocolate chips (optional)

½ tsp baking powder

> Whisk eggs, melted butter or oil, vanilla, coconut nectar, and salt together.
> Add flour, cacao powder, baking powder, and chocolate chips.
> Grease brownie dish with coconut oil and bake at 350 for 10-15 minutes.
> Serves 8.

Lemon Chia Seed Scones

2 cups almond flour

½ cup coconut flour

2 pastured eggs

⅓ cup coconut sugar

10 drops lemon essential oil

2 Tbsp chia seeds

> Mix eggs, flours, coconut sugar, essential oil, and chia seeds together.
> Form into cookies/scones and bake at 350 for 15 minutes.
> Serves 8-12.

Walnut Scones

2 ½ cups almond flour

4 Tbsp coconut flour

½ tsp baking soda

⅓ cup coconut sugar

⅔ cup melted coconut oil

3 pastured eggs

1 Tbsp vanilla extract

⅔ cup walnut halves

> Combine almond flour, coconut flour, baking soda, and coconut sugar.
> Whisk together oil, eggs, and vanilla.
> Pour wet ingredients into dry ingredients.
> Fold in walnuts.
> Bake at 350 for 10 minutes.
> Variations: Add almond extract in place of vanilla and almonds in place of walnuts.
> Serves 8.

Lemon Pound Cake

6 pastured eggs

1 cup grass-fed butter, melted

⅓ cup raw, unheated honey

7 drops lemon essential oil

½ tsp sea salt

½ cup coconut flour

1 tsp baking powder

> Blend together eggs, butter/ghee, honey, lemon essential oil, and salt. Add in coconut flour and baking powder, whisk thoroughly into batter until there are no lumps. Pour into greased loaf/bread pan. Bake at 325 degrees for 20-30 minutes. Let it cool for 45-60 minutes before serving.
> Serves 6.

Almond Bliss

½ cup raw coconut butter

½ cup raw almonds

4 dark chocolate bars

⅓ cup coconut flakes

> Place two almonds in each candy mold.
> Warm coconut butter and spoon onto almonds (a Tbsp at a time).
> Melt chocolate and spoon on top of coconut butter.
> Sprinkle with coconut flakes.
> Freeze and serve cold.
> Serves 8.

Fig Cookies

2 ½ cups almond flour

2 Tbsp coconut flour

½ tsp sea salt

½ cup melted coconut oil

⅓ cup maple syrup

⅓ cup raw, unheated honey

1 Tbsp vanilla extract

FIG FILLING:

1 ½ cups figs

¼ cup fresh lemon juice

1 Tbsp vanilla extract

> Whisk melted oil, maple syrup, honey, and vanilla together.
> Pour into flours and salt and mix well.
> Place in the fridge for 1 hour.

> FIG FILLING: Pulse ingredients in a high-speed blender or food processor until it is a paste.
> Roll out fig cookie "crust" and cut into square shapes.
> Spread fig "paste" over half the crust.
> Fold the crust over it like a tortilla.
> With fingers, press down the edges of the dough.
> Bake at 350 for 10 minutes.
> Serves 12.

Baked Pears in Caramel Sauce

6 medium-sized pears, peeled and cored

½ cup maple syrup

½ cup unsalted grass-fed butter

1 ¼ cup whipped coconut cream or Amasai mixed with raw, unheated honey

1 tsp vanilla extract

¼ tsp cardamom

> Cut pears in half lengthwise and put in lightly greased glass baking dish. Melt butter in saucepan. Add maple syrup and whisk until combined well. Pour over pear halves. Bake at 400 degrees for 30 minutes.

> In separate bowl, add whipped coconut cream or Amasai, vanilla, and cardamom. Whisk thoroughly and pour evenly over pears. Bake an additional 15 minutes, basting pears with creamy mixture. Serve warm.

> Serves 6.

Mocha Coco Cookies

½ cup coconut oil

¾ cup coconut sugar

4 pastured eggs

½ tsp vanilla extract

½ cup coconut flour

2 cups unsweetened coconut flakes

1 cup dark chocolate chips

> Mix eggs, coconut sugar, coconut oil, and vanilla together in a mixer.

> Add coconut flour and flakes.

> Mix well.

> Drop by spoonfuls on a pan and form into cookies.

> Bake at 375 for 15-20 minutes.

> Melt chocolate chips over the stove and drizzle over cookie.

> Serves 8.

Grain Free Apple Pie

4 apples, sliced

½ cup coconut sugar

¼ cup maple syrup (optional)

½ cup water

2 Tbsp arrowroot powder

½ cup raisins

1 tsp cinnamon

½ tsp nutmeg

1 tsp vanilla

1 grain free pie crust (see recipe below)

CRUMBLE TOPPING:

¾ cup pecans

1 tsp cinnamon

⅓ cup coconut sugar

GRAIN FREE PIE CRUST:

1 ½ cups almond flour

1 pastured egg

1 Tbsp raw, unheated honey

½ tsp sea salt

> In a pot, place sliced apples and ½ cup of water.
> Turn the stove on low and place the cover on.
> Let the apples cook for a good 10 minutes until soft.
> Add arrowroot powder, first mixing it in about ¼ cup of water.
> Add coconut sugar, syrup, cinnamon, nutmeg, raisins, and vanilla.
> Stir around until mixture has thickened.
> Pour into pie crust and add crumble topping.
> Bake at 350 for 5-10 minutes.

> GRAIN FREE PIE CRUST: Mix all ingredients together.
> Grease pie pan/tin with coconut oil.
> Roll out dough and place in the pie pan.
> Bake at 350 for 5 minutes.
> Take out and let cool before adding filling.
> Serve at room temperature.
> Serves 8.

Rainbow Fruit with Mango Cream

1 cup blackberries

1 cup mango, peeled, pitted, and diced

1 cup strawberries, diced

1 cup blueberries

MANGO CREAM:

½ cup coconut cream (the heavy cream on top of the coconut milk can)

3 ripe mangos, peeled, pitted, and sliced

½ of a medium ripe banana

1 Tbsp raw, unheated honey or pure maple syrup

> In a clear goblet, layer ¼ cup of blueberries, ¼ cup diced mango, ¼ cup strawberries, and ¼ cup blueberries. Refrigerate until ready to serve. Just before serving, put a generous dollop of mango cream on top of fruit in each glass.

> MANGO CREAM: Refrigerate the can of coconut milk overnight so that the heavy cream rises to the top. Scoop off ½ cup. In a mixing bowl, with electric mixer, whip coconut cream until stiff.

> Blend mangos, banana, and maple syrup or honey in blender or food processor until smooth. Fold into whipped coconut cream. Refrigerate at least one hour. Serve on top of fruit goblets.

> Serves 4.

Snowballs

4 Tbsp ground chia seeds

2 Tbsp coconut flour

¼ cup raw cacao powder

1 Tbsp raw, unheated honey

⅓-½ cup coconut oil

1 tsp vanilla extract

½ cup coconut shreds

½ tsp sea salt

> Mix ground chia, raw cacao, and coconut flour together.

> Add honey, coconut oil, vanilla, and salt.

> Form into balls and roll in coconut shreds.

> Freeze or place in the fridge for an hour and serve cool.

main
dishes

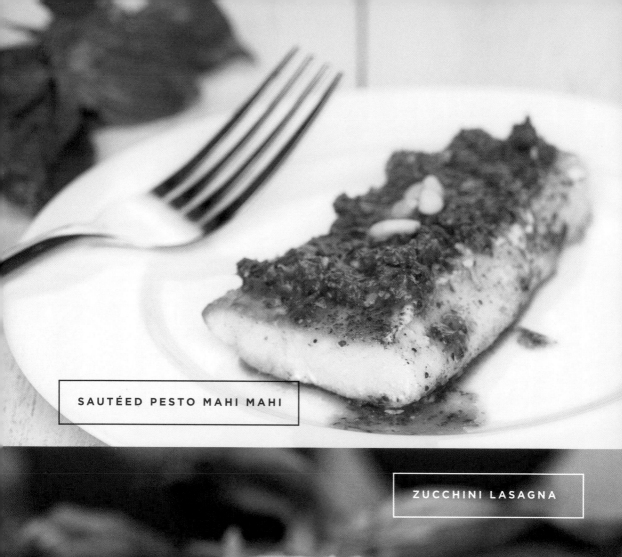

SAUTÉED PESTO MAHI MAHI

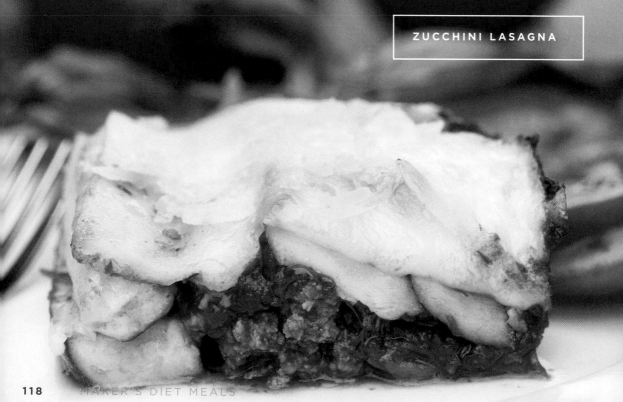

ZUCCHINI LASAGNA

MAKER'S DIET MEALS

Sautéed Pesto Mahi Mahi

4 Mahi Mahi fish fillets, fresh or frozen

1 lemon

PESTO:

2 cups fresh basil, sage, cilantro, and parsley, lightly packed

2 cloves garlic

½ cup olive oil

¼ cup pine nuts

½ cup green-fed raw cheese, grated

> Place all pesto ingredients, except the cheese, in your food processor and process until the mixture is creamy. Toss in the cheese and pulse.

> Heat a heavy skillet until just starting to smoke over medium-high heat. Add coconut oil. Rub fish on both sides with the pesto mixture. Sauté in pan until fish flakes easily, approximately 3-5 minutes per side.

> When fish is done, brush both sides with pesto sauce again. Squeeze lemon over the fish and serve immediately.

> Serves 4.

Zucchini Lasagna

2 ½ lbs grass-fed ground beef

1 red onion, diced

4 cloves garlic, crushed

2 Tbsp dried oregano

2 Tbsp dried basil

½ tsp cayenne pepper

½ tsp sea salt

2 Tbsp olive oil

3 cups tomatoes, diced

6 ounces tomato paste

1 cup black olives, sliced

6 zucchinis, thinly sliced

1 cup green-fed cheddar or goat cheese

> In a large pot, sauté onions and garlic in the olive oil for 3 minutes.

> Add ground beef and sausage and brown. Add in all dry ingredients. Mix in diced tomatoes and tomato paste.

> In a big lasagna baking dish, place a layer of sliced zucchini and then ladle on a thick layer of the meat mixture and top with the sliced black olives.

> Top meat and olive layer with another layer of sliced zucchini and top with a final layer of the remaining meat mixture. Top with shredded cheese. Cover tightly with aluminum foil.

> Bake at 350 degrees for 30 min.

> Serves 4.

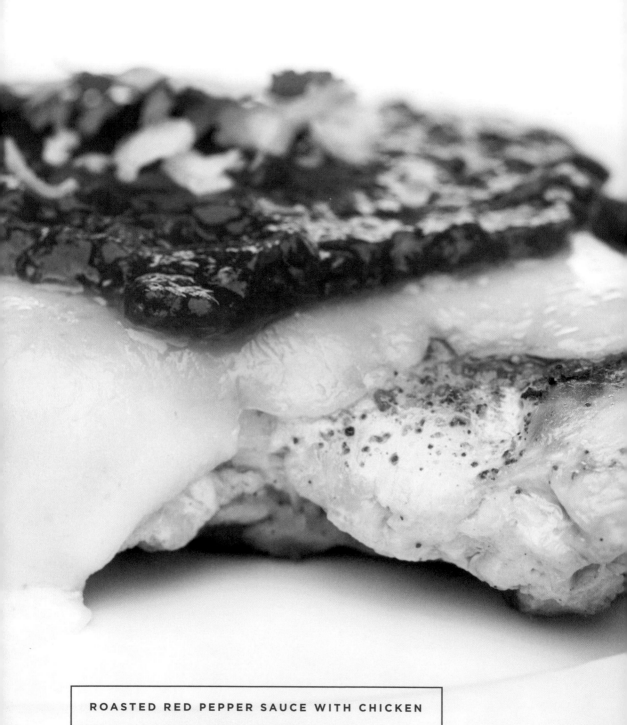

ROASTED RED PEPPER SAUCE WITH CHICKEN

Roasted Red Pepper Sauce with Chicken

4 boneless, skinless chicken breasts

4 slices green-fed, raw cheddar cheese

1 red bell pepper

¼ cup olive oil

2 garlic cloves, minced

½ tsp onion powder

¼ tsp cayenne pepper

½ tsp sea salt

½ tsp thyme

> Line a baking sheet with foil. Cut bell pepper into medium-sized strips and place on the prepared baking sheet. Drizzle with the ¼ cup olive oil. Bake for 10 minutes at 500 degrees.

> Place peppers in blender along with garlic cloves, onion powder, cayenne pepper, sea salt, and thyme. Blend until smooth, approximately 1 minute.

> Sauté chicken with coconut oil and season with salt and pepper.

> Place cheese on each chicken breast, return to skillet and cover until cheese melts. Spoon a few tablespoons of red pepper sauce over chicken.

> Serves about 4.

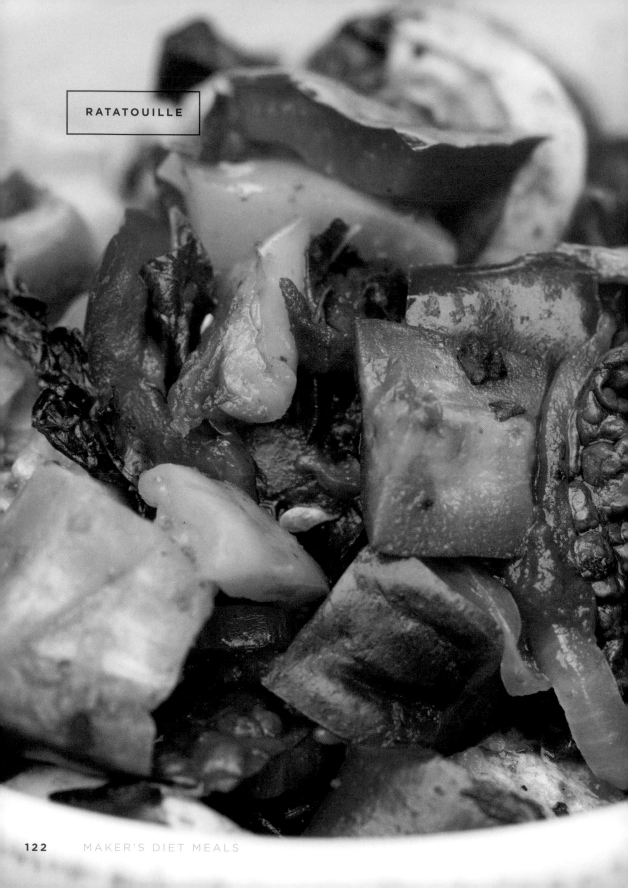

RATATOUILLE

Ratatouille

¼ cup melted grass-fed butter, plus more as needed

1 ½ cups small diced yellow onion

1 tsp minced garlic

2 cups medium diced eggplant, skin on

½ tsp fresh thyme leaves

1 cup diced green bell peppers

1 cup diced red bell peppers

1 cup diced zucchini squash

1 cup diced yellow squash

1 ½ cups peeled, seeded, and chopped tomatoes

1 Tbsp thinly sliced fresh basil leaves

1 Tbsp chopped fresh parsley leaves

Salt and freshly ground black pepper

> Set a large sauté pan over medium heat and add the butter. Once hot, add the onions and garlic to the pan. Cook the onions, stirring occasionally, until they are wilted and lightly caramelized, about 5-7 minutes.

> Add the eggplant and thyme to the pan and continue to cook, stirring occasionally, until the eggplant is partially cooked, about 5 minutes.

> Add the green and red peppers, zucchini, and squash, and continue to cook for an additional 5 minutes.

> Add the tomatoes, basil, parsley, and salt and pepper to taste, and cook for a final 5 minutes.

> Stir well to blend and serve either hot or at room temperature.

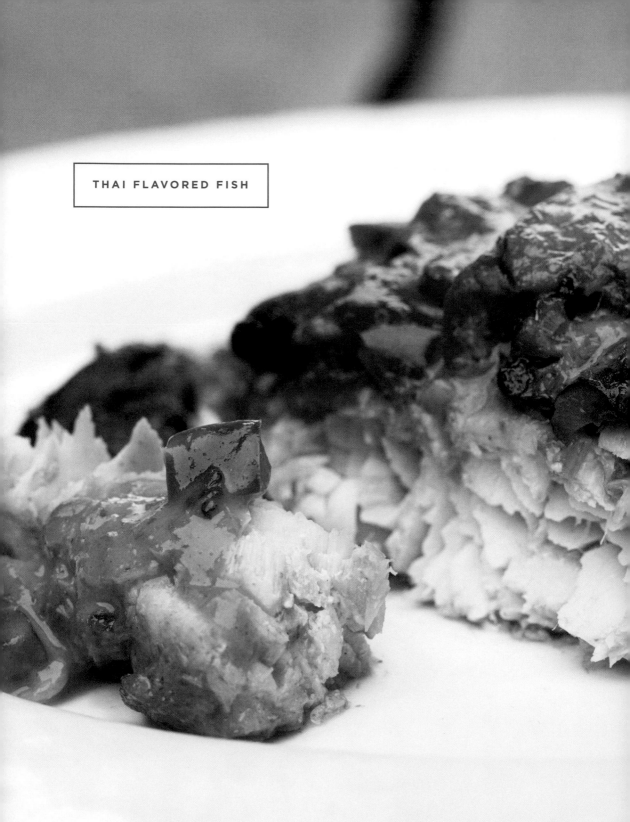

THAI FLAVORED FISH

Thai Flavored Fish

FISH:

4 fillets wild-caught white fish, such as mahi mahi or cod

2 Tbsp coconut oil

2 tsp paprika

½ tsp onion powder

¼ tsp garlic powder

Sea salt and pepper to season

> FISH: Combine all spices and rub into fillets. Heat coconut oil over medium-high heat and cook fillets until they are cooked through and flake easily, turning once.

> Serve with sauce over quinoa.

FISH SAUCE:

2 Tbsp coconut oil

1 shallot, finely minced

1 ½ cup baby portobello mushrooms, sliced

½ cup red bell pepper, diced

2 Tbsp lemongrass paste

1 tsp Thai red curry paste

1 - 1 ½ tsp chili pepper

1 tsp Worcestershire sauce

6 Tbsp coconut milk

> FISH SAUCE: Sauté the shallot, mushrooms, and red bell pepper in coconut oil in skillet over medium heat.

> While mushroom mixture is cooking, mix lemongrass paste, curry paste, chili pepper paste, Worcestershire, and coconut milk in a small bowl. When mushrooms are done and onion is transparent, add the curry paste mixture to your skillet and stir well.

> Serves 4.

BLACK BEAN CHILI

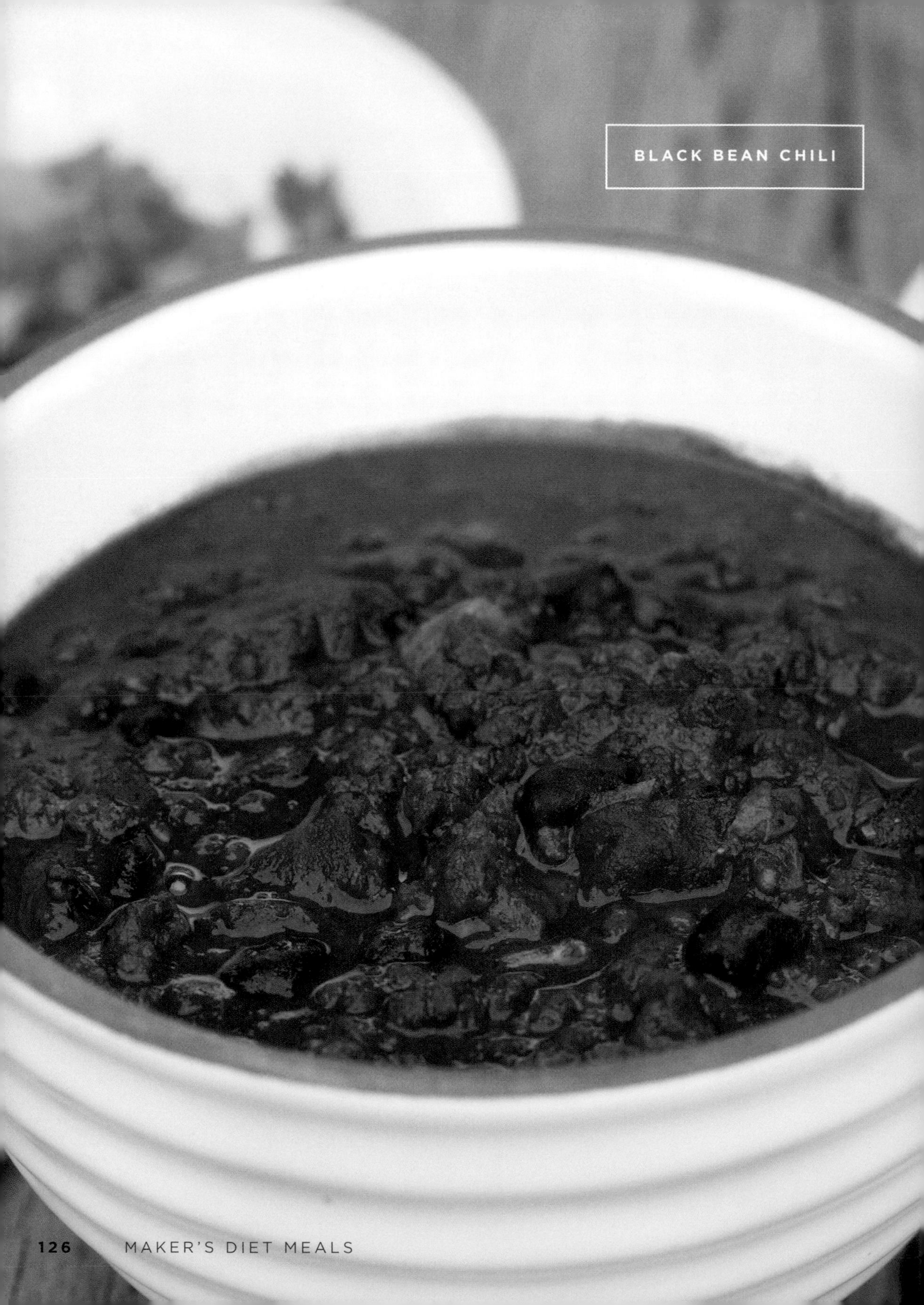

Black Bean Chili

6 Tbsp coconut oil

3 lbs grass-fed beef, cut into half inch chunks or ground

2 large onions, chopped

2 large carrots, peeled and diced

8 cloves garlic, chopped

1 jalapeno pepper, seeded and finely chopped

3 Tbsp whole spelt flour

¼ cup chili powder

1 ½ Tbsp dried cumin

1 Tbsp dried oregano

1 tsp dried cinnamon

2 tsp sea salt

¼ tsp red pepper flakes

5 cups beef broth

1 28-oz can organic plum tomatoes, drained and chopped

1 28-oz can organic crushed tomatoes

2 chipotle chilies in adobo sauce

2 15-oz cans black beans

½ ounce (half of a square) unsweetened dark chocolate, grated

1 cup green-fed, raw cheddar cheese or goat cheese, shredded

1 cup organic sour cream

½ cup cilantro, chopped

Corn or multigrain tortilla chips

> In a large, deep, heavy dutch oven, heat 2 tablespoons of oil over medium heat. Cook the meat in 2 batches, turning often, until browned on all sides. Add more oil as necessary. Transfer the meat to a bowl.

> Add 2 more tablespoons of oil and cook the onions, carrots, and garlic until softened, about 2 or 3 minutes. Return the browned meat to the pot.

> Sprinkle the meat and vegetable mixture with the flour and stir and cook for 1 minute.

> Add the chili powder, cumin, oregano, cinnamon, salt, red pepper flakes, tomatoes, and beef broth.

> If you have latex gloves, you might want to put them on. You are going to add a couple of the chipotle chilies from the can that you have. These are very, very hot! I removed the seeds from one of them and chopped it and put it in the chili. I put in the other one whole and fished it out when the chili was done. If you like your chili spicy, add the whole can but be warned, they are HOT!!! The adobo sauce is wonderfully smoky, so add about a tablespoon of that from the can.

> Simmer partially covered over low heat for about 1 to 1 ½ hours or until the meat is tender and the chili has cooked down. You want it thick, but not too thick. Stir it occasionally. It will probably stick a bit on the bottom. That's okay, just make sure your heat isn't on too high.

> Open two cans of black beans, drain them, and add them to the chili. Grate the chocolate and add it as well. Taste and adjust seasonings if needed.

> Serve garnished with cheese, chopped cilantro, Amasai, chopped jalapenos, and tortilla chips. Enjoy!

> Serves 6-8.

BUTTERNUT SQUASH BAKE

CHEDDAR AND BEEF CASSEROLE

Butternut Squash Bake

1 butternut squash

1 red onion, chopped

1 zucchini, chopped

½ cup grass-fed butter

> Chop all ingredients.
> In large bowl, mix together with butter.
> Bake at 450 degrees for 15-20 minutes in oven.
> Serves 4.

Cheddar and Beef Casserole

10 pastured eggs

1 lb. grass-fed ground beef

8 oz plain Amasai or sheep milk yogurt

6 oz grass-fed, raw cheddar cheese or goat cheese, shredded (2 cups)

½ tsp sea salt

1 tsp nutmeg

½ tsp black pepper

> Whisk eggs, Amasai, nutmeg, pepper, and salt together.
> Spread the ground beef evenly in a greased baking dish (greased with coconut oil).
> Pour eggs over the beef.
> Sprinkle the cheese evenly on top.
> Bake at 350 degrees for 15-20 minutes.

GRILLED FRUIT STEAK

CREAMY CUCUMBER AVOCADO SOUP

Grilled Fruit Steak

6 oz grass-fed steak

1 avocado

1 mango

1 pineapple

> Slice fruit.
> Place fruit and steak on grill.
> Grill fruit on each side for 5 minutes.
> Grill steak on each side for 10 minutes.
> Sprinkle black pepper over top of fruit and steak.
> Serves 1.

Creamy Cucumber Avocado Soup

½ cucumber

1 ripe avocado

5 stalks celery

3 Tbsp lemon juice

½ cup cultured whey

1 tsp sea salt

½ tsp black pepper

2 oz green-fed, raw cheddar cheese or goat cheese

> Blend all ingredients (except the cheese) together in a high powered blender.
> Serve chilled with cheese (either on the side or on top).
> Serves 4.

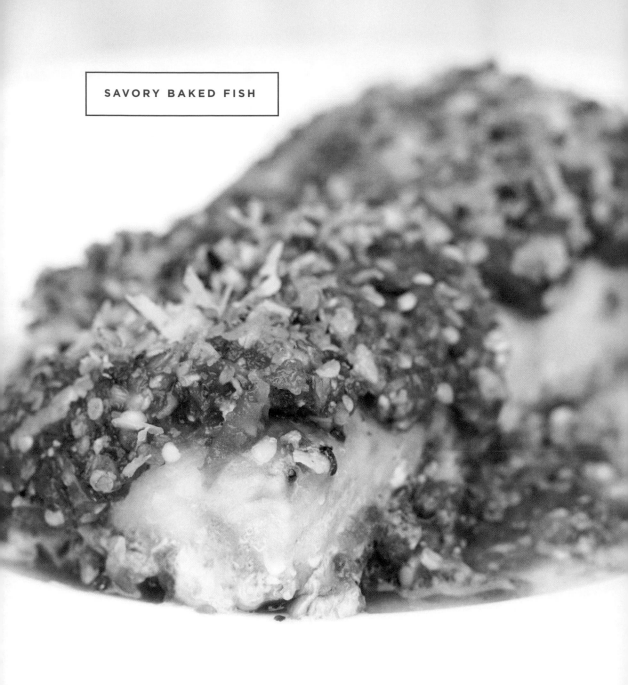

SAVORY BAKED FISH

Savory Baked Fish

6 fillets of white fish, such as mahi mahi, grouper, or snapper

Sea salt and freshly ground pepper to taste

3 cloves garlic, finely minced

½ cup onion, finely minced

3 Tbsp extra virgin olive oil

1 tsp onion powder

1 tsp lemon pepper seasoning

½ tsp celery salt

½ tsp paprika

1 8-oz can fire roasted diced tomatoes

4 Tbsp Italian parsley, chopped

1 Tbsp Terrain Fermented Kombucha or apple cider vinegar

3 Tbsp grated aged green-fed, raw Havarti cheese

3 Tbsp almond flour or bread crumbs (from toasted whole grain sourdough bread)

> Sauté the onions and garlic in the olive oil in a small skillet over medium-low until onion is transparent and soft. Puree fire roasted tomatoes in blender. Add garlic/onion mix to blender with tomatoes and other herbs.

> Place fish in baking pan that has been coated with olive oil. Generously brush fish with tomato sauce mixture.

> In a small bowl, mix flour and cheese together. Sprinkle cheese mixture over fish and bake at 350 degrees for approximately 30 minutes.

> Serves 6.

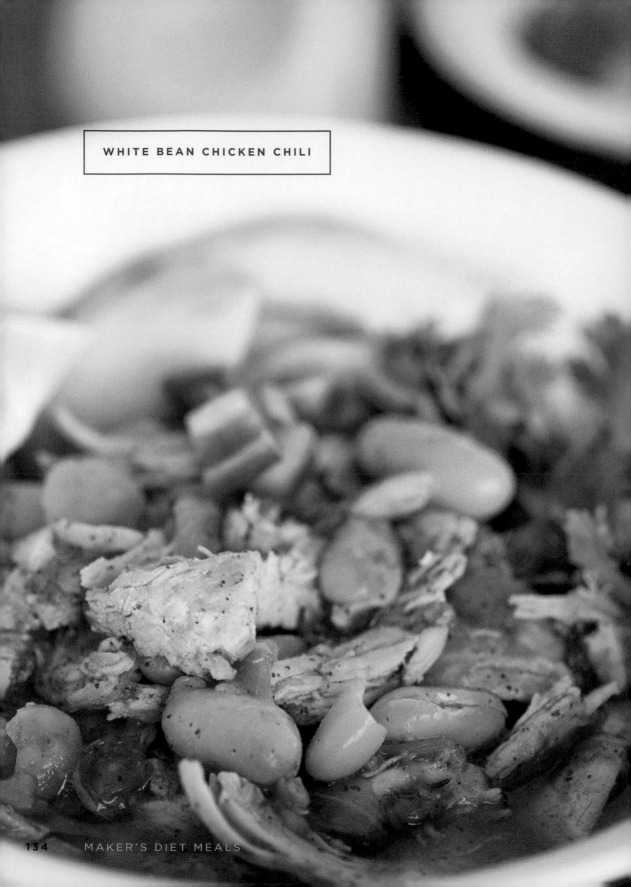

WHITE BEAN CHICKEN CHILI

White Bean Chicken Chili

3-4 cups pasture-raised chicken, shredded

3 Tbsp coconut

Sea salt and pepper

1 onion, chopped

3 cloves garlic, chopped

2 jalapeno peppers, seeded and de-ribbed, then chopped

4 ounce can of chopped green chilies

1 tsp dried oregano

¼ tsp ground cayenne

1 Tbsp chili powder

2-3 cups chicken broth

1 can white or pinto beans

Garnishes: avocado, chopped; lime, sliced; one cup grated green-fed, raw cheese; one cup plain Amasai or sheep milk yogurt

TIPS:

- Jalapenos when cooked lose a lot of their heat if you remove the ribs and seeds. No matter what, use rubber or plastic gloves when chopping them. You don't want to get jalapeno juice in your eyes!

- You can switch up the spices if you like. Cumin or coriander would both be good choices.

- I use cannelini beans, but you can really use any beans you like. Even black beans.

- To stretch this even further, use two cans of beans.

- Crumble tortilla chips on top for a nice crunch.

> Roast the chicken breasts. Preheat oven to 350, rinse and dry chicken breasts and coat with one tablespoon of the oil, then sprinkle with salt and pepper. Place on a rimmed baking sheet and roast for about 40 minutes. The skin will be crisp and beginning to brown. I save all the bones and skin and use it to make homemade stock.

> Remove chicken from oven and let it cool. Shred it or chop the meat when cool enough to handle.

> Sauté the chopped onion and garlic in 2 Tbsp of oil for about 3 minutes.

> Add the chopped jalapeno and sauté for an additional three minutes.

> Add the spices and let it all cook about 2 minutes to allow the flavors to blend.

> Add the chicken broth, beans, and shredded chicken and simmer for about 20 minutes. Some of the liquid should evaporate as you don't want it soupy. If it gets too dry, add more broth.

> While it's simmering, chop an avocado, slice a lime, grate some raw cheddar or goat cheese and scoop out some Amasai.

> Serve in bowls and pass the garnishes.

> Serves 6.

SPINACH CHICKEN ROLL

Spinach Chicken Roll

3 Tbsp butter

4 Tbsp garlic, minced

6 cups packed fresh spinach

7 oz can artichoke hearts, rinsed and drained, rough chopped

½ cup sun-dried tomatoes, chopped

½ cup grated raw green-fed aged Havarti cheese

½ cup green-fed, raw cheddar cheese or goat cheese

6 boneless skinless pasture-raised chicken breasts

Sea salt and pepper to taste

> Melt the butter in a medium-sized skillet and add in garlic and spinach. In other skillet, add artichokes and cook over medium heat, then add all other ingredients. Stir until everything is well combined and starting to blend together, including garlic and spinach.

> Put approximately 2 rounded tablespoons of the spinach mixture at the end of each chicken breast. Roll the chicken breasts up and gently tuck the ends in to help keep the spinach mixture in during cooking. Secure with toothpicks. Sprinkle with salt and pepper.

> Bake chicken for 15 minutes at 400 or fry in pan with coconut oil.

> Serves 6.

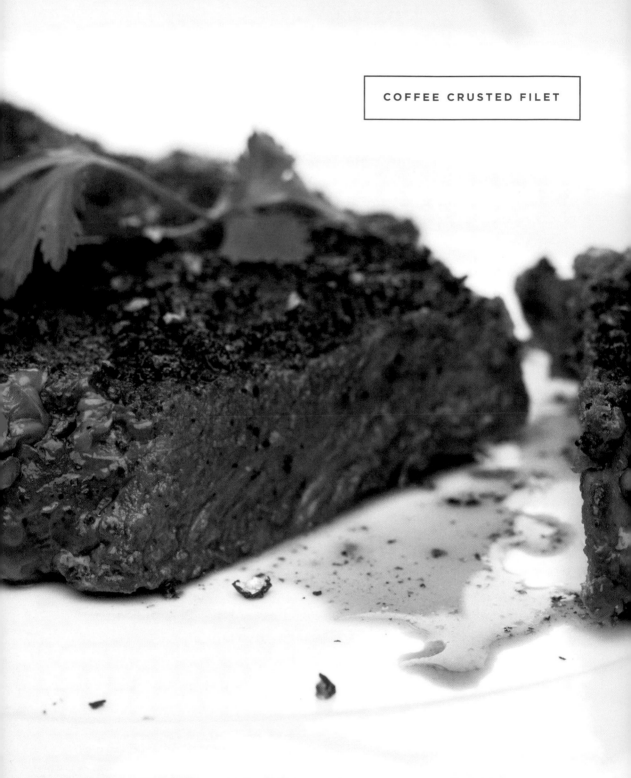

COFFEE CRUSTED FILET

Coffee Crusted Filet

4 grass-fed tenderloins

½ cup of medium roast coffee beans (grind yourself)

2 Tbsp fresh ground pepper

¼ cup coconut sugar

2 Tbsp sea salt

2 Tbsp granulated garlic

1 ½ Tbsp paprika

½ Tbsp cayenne pepper

1 tsp onion powder

½ tsp thyme

6 Tbsp grass-fed butter

> Combine coffee, pepper, coconut sugar, salt, garlic, cayenne pepper, paprika, onion powder, and thyme in a bowl. Stir thoroughly. Rub coffee mixture toughly into both sides of the beef fillets.

> Prepare a cast iron skillet by heating the butter in skillet until it is very hot and almost smoking. Add the steaks and sear on both sides for about 3 minutes each side and a nice brown crust forms. Remove the skillet from the fire and put in oven at 400 degrees for 6 minutes.

> Serves 4.

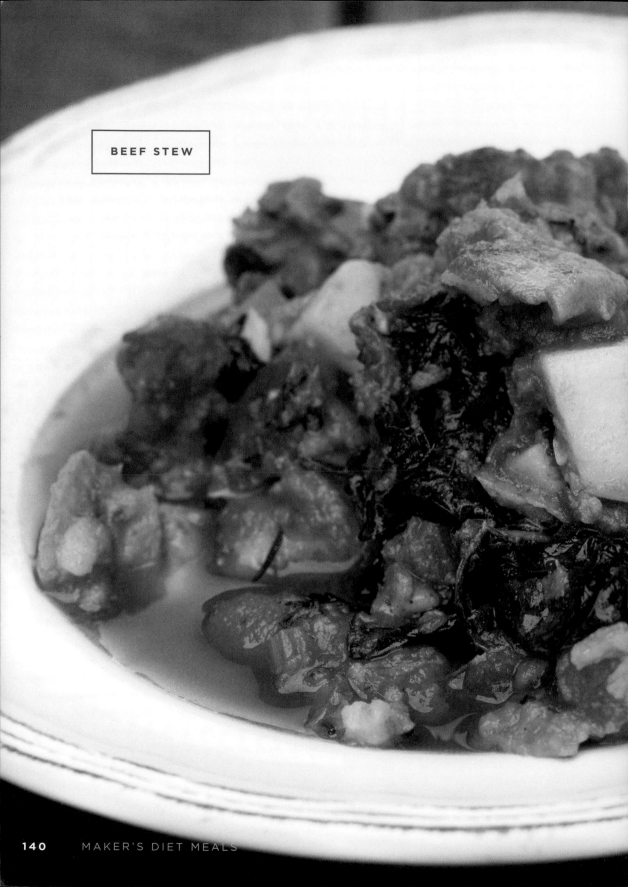

BEEF STEW

Beef Stew

2 lbs. grass-fed beef stew meat

2 Tbsp olive oil

1 cup celery, diced

3 garlic cloves, minced

1 medium onion, diced

1 sprig fresh thyme

1 sprig fresh rosemary

1 Tbsp Worcestershire sauce

1 cup mini carrots

1 can (14.5 oz) fireroasted tomatoes, diced

1 Tbsp coconut sugar

1 tsp sea salt

½ tsp pepper

3 sweet potatoes, cubed

½ cup beef broth

> Put all ingredients in crockpot and cook for 4-8 hours.

> Serves 4-6.

CASHEW CHICKEN WITH APRICOT SAUCE

CHICKEN VEGGIE SOUP

Cashew Chicken with Apricot Sauce

1 cup dried apricots,
(no sulfites)

6 medjool dates

1 ½ cup boiling water

2 Tbsp raw, unheated honey

2 Tbsp dijon mustard

1 cup coarsely chopped cashews

1 ¼ tsp curry powder

4 boneless, skinless pasture-raised chicken breasts

Sea salt and freshly ground pepper to taste

> Cover baking dish with coconut oil. In medium bowl, soak the apricots and dates in the hot water for at least 1 hour.

> In the food processor, blend soaked apricots, dates, and honey until thick. Add the mustard and curry powder and pulse until thoroughly blended. Pour the sauce in bowl, then add cashews.

> Dip chicken breasts in the apricot mixture, coating well. Roll coated chicken breasts in nuts and place in baking dish. Bake in oven at 375 degrees for 25-30 minutes.

> Serves 4.

Chicken Veggie Soup

32 oz homemade bone broth

5 cups chopped veggies (mushroom, celery, broccoli, carrot, onion)

6 oz free range chicken (cut with kitchen scissors)

3 cloves garlic

1 tsp salt

½ tsp black pepper

1 Tbsp basil

1 cup shredded raw, green-fed cheddar cheese

> Simmer all ingredients in large pot (except cheese).

> Add cheese after soup is done.

Chicken with Mushroom Wine Sauce

4 boneless skinless pasture-raised chicken breasts

SAUCE:

4 Tbsp grass-fed unsalted butter

2 Tbsp fresh parsley, minced

1 large garlic clove, finely minced

4 green onions, sliced thinly, white and green parts

2 cups chicken broth

¼ tsp nutmeg

1 Tbsp tapioca flour

1 ¼ cups fresh mushrooms, sliced

1 cup dry sherry

> Flatten chicken to ¼ inch. Season to taste and grill over indirect heat on gas or charcoal until chicken is fully cooked.

> Melt butter in medium skillet over medium-low heat. Add onions, mushrooms, and garlic and cook, stirring constantly until onion begins to be transparent. Mix chicken broth and tapioca flour together in a small bowl then add to skillet. Add parsley and nutmeg. Stir.

> Simmer for about 15 minutes. Add the sherry and bring to a boil. Boil for 1 minute. Serve over cooked chicken breasts.

> Serves 4.

Lemon Grilled Chicken Legs

8 pasture-raised chicken legs

½ cup grass-fed butter

⅔ cup fresh squeezed lemon juice

Zest from three lemons

2 large garlic cloves, finely minced

1 tsp paprika

½ tsp cayenne pepper

1 sprig fresh oregano

1 sprig fresh rosemary

1 tsp sea salt

½ tsp black pepper

> Melt butter in small saucepan. Take off heat and add rest of the ingredients. Marinate chicken in glass dish overnight to at least 4-5 hours before grilling. Turn once or twice during the marinating time. Grill chicken until done.

> Serves 4-6

Moroccan Chicken Skewers

2 red bell peppers, cut into 1 inch cubes

20 small mushrooms

2 medium red onions, cut into 1 inch cubes

½ tsp ground ginger

2 tsp paprika

½ tsp turmeric

2 garlic cloves, crushed

3 Tbsp fresh cilantro, chopped

2 Tbsp fresh parsley, chopped

1 ½ Tbsp fresh squeezed lemon juice

1 ½ Tbsp extra virgin olive oil

1 ½ lbs pasture-raised chicken breasts, cut into 1 inch cubes

Sea salt and pepper to taste

> Mix all herbs, juice, and oil together. Coat chicken cubes with mixture. Cover and let marinate in refrigerator overnight.

> Alternate chicken cubes, peppers, lemon chunks, and onions on skewers. Cook 6-7 minutes on each side. Serve with quinoa or brown rice.

> Serves 5-6.

Chicken Nuggets

2 large pastured chicken breasts

1 cup coconut flour

2 pastured eggs

1 Tbsp garlic powder

1 tsp sea salt

1 tsp dried basil

1 tsp dried oregano

1 Tbsp ghee

1 Tbsp coconut oil

> Place chicken on a plate or cutting board and slice into strips.

> Dip into egg.

> Dip into flour and herbs.

> Sprinkle with salt and cook.

> Serves 4.

Meatballs

1 lb grass-fed ground beef

1 pastured egg

2 Tbsp coconut flour

1 Tbsp dried basil

1 Tbsp dried oregano

1 tsp sea salt

SAUCE:

1 can tomato paste

1 Tbsp dried basil

1 Tbsp dried oregano

1 tsp sea salt

½ cup water

1 clove of minced garlic
(optional)

> Mix all ingredients together.
> Form into meatballs.
> Cook in coconut oil until done.
> Add sauce and cover to keep warm.

> SAUCE: Mix all ingredients together in a bowl.
> Pour over meatballs.
> Top with green-fed raw cheddar cheese or goat cheese.
> Serves 3.

Sausage and Bean Casserole

2 Tbsp olive oil

grass-fed beef, turkey, or chicken sausage

1 large onion, chopped

2 garlic cloves, minced

2 large carrots, thinly sliced

1 cup red wine

2 cans fire roasted tomatoes, diced

2 cans Great Northern beans

2 Tbsp red wine vinegar

1 tsp raw, unheated honey

2 Tbsp fresh parsley, finely chopped

> On medium heat, warm coconut oil. Cook sausages and carrots until sausages are nicely browned all over. Put sausage mixture into a separate dish or bowl and set aside.

> In the same Dutch oven add garlic and onions and cook until transparent. Add the wine, tomatoes, and beans. Simmer for about 5 minutes. Return sausages and carrots to pan and lower heat to simmer for 15 minutes. Add red wine vinegar, parsley, and honey. Stir well. Simmer 2 more minutes and then serve.

> Serves 6-8.

Asian Chicken Stir Fry

4 cups shredded carrots

4 cups broccoli

2 cups peas

8 oz pastured chicken
(precooked)

1 cup unpasteurized soy sauce
or coconut aminos

2 Tbsp dried ginger

3 drops orange essential oil

2 Tbsp coconut oil

> Melt coconut oil in a large skillet on
  low heat.

> Place all ingredients in, except the
  orange essential oil and chicken.

> Cook for 30 minutes on low heat.

> Add orange oil and chicken and
  cook for 5 to 10 more minutes.

> Serves 5.

Zucchini Mushroom Stir Fry

4 cups mushrooms

4 cups chopped zucchini

2 cups chopped sweet onion

4 cups spinach

3 Tbsp clarified butter (ghee)

1 cup green-fed, raw cheddar
cheese or goat cheese

> Melt ghee in a large skillet on low.

> Place onions in and let it sauté for
  10-15 minutes.

> Add remaining ingredients except
  cheese and sauté for 30 minutes.

> Add cheese and turn off stove.

> Serves 5.

Healthy Veggie Burger

1 cup cooked quinoa

1 cup sweet potato, peeled and finely diced

½ cup onion, minced

16 oz can black beans, rinsed and drained well

3 cloves garlic, minced

1 Tbsp chili powder

2 tsp ground cumin

½ tsp sea salt

½ tsp pepper

1 pastured egg, well beaten

GARLIC AOLI:

½ cup mayonnaise

2 cloves garlic, finely minced

2 Tbsp freshly squeezed lemon juice

¼ tsp dijon mustard

½ tsp salt

¼ tsp black pepper

> Mix all ingredients together in bowl. Cook over medium heat in coconut oil.

> Serve the veggie burger on a bed of lettuce with a lightly toasted, whole grain bun. Top one side of the bun with the garlic aoli and the other side with guacamole. Add sliced tomato, lettuce, thinly sliced onion, and pickle if desired.

> GARLIC AOLI: Mix all ingredients well and refrigerate for 1 hour to give flavors time to blend.

> Serves 5.

Surf and Turf Kabobs

2 pieces of wild-caught white fish, such as mahi mahi, cod, or halibut

8 oz green-fed sirloin or fillet beef, cut into one inch cubes

2 large sweet potatoes, cut into one inch cubes

1 cup pineapple juice

2 large red or orange bell pepper, cut into one inch cubes

10 medium-sized button mushrooms

1 fresh pineapple, cut into one inch chunks

Sea salt and pepper to taste

12 metal skewers

MARINADE:

Juice and zest of 2 lemons

1 Tbsp Terrain Fermented Turmeric or 1 tsp dried turmeric powder

3 cloves garlic, finely minced

½ teaspoon cayenne pepper

½ cup onion, finely minced

4 Tbsp unpasteurized soy sauce or coconut aminos

4 Tbsp raw, unheated honey

2 tsp minced ginger root

Pinch of freshly ground black pepper

> Thoroughly mix all ingredients in a medium-sized glass bowl. Divide marinade in half and put in separate glass bowls. Marinate the beef cubes in one bowl for 3-6 hours and refrigerate. One hour before grilling, marinate fish cubes, peppers, and mushrooms in the second glass container in refrigerator.

> Boil the sweet potato cubes in the pineapple juice until just tender, but not falling apart. When sweet potatoes are cool enough to touch, thread the skewers. Arrange one piece of each: fish, sweet potato, bell pepper, beef, pineapple, and mushroom.

> Cook kabobs, turning as needed.

> Serves 6.

Fish Tacos with Mango Salsa

1 pound firm wild fish, such as mahi mahi or cod

¼ cup olive oil

1 lime, juiced

1 Tbsp ancho chili powder

½ tsp granulated garlic

Sprouted corn or grain tortillas

MANGO/AVOCADO SALSA

1 ripe avocado, pitted and cut in small cubes

1 ripe mango, pitted and cut in small cubes

½ cup red bell pepper, minced

1 jalapeño pepper, seeded and diced

1 Tbsp fresh lime juice

2 Tbsp fresh cilantro, finely chopped

1 Tbsp fresh parsley, finely chopped

1 tsp coconut sugar

> Preheat grill to medium-high heat. Place fish in a medium-sized dish. Whisk together the oil, lime juice, garlic, ancho, and cilantro and pour over fish. Let marinate for 20 minutes.

> Cook for 4-5 minutes or until fish flakes easily when tested with a fork.

> Serve with toppings of shredded cabbage, sliced green onion, chopped cilantro, and mango avocado salsa.

> Serves 6.

> MANGO/AVOCADO SALSA: Combine all ingredients together and stir well. Refrigerate until ready to serve.

Maple Glazed Sausage Kabobs

½ pound fully cooked grass-fed beef summer sausage

1 red onion, cut into 1-inch cubes

4 apricots, plums, or peaches, cut in half

1 sweet red pepper, seeded and cut into chunks

¼ cup maple syrup

2 Tbsp whole grain mustard

1 Tbsp unpasteurized soy sauce or coconut aminos

1 Tbsp Worcestershire sauce

1 tsp crushed dried rosemary leaves

1 tsp dried thyme

2 tsp smoked chipotle peppers, minced

7-8 metal skewers

> Stir together maple syrup, mustard, soy sauce, Worcestershire sauce, thyme, rosemary, and chipotle pepper. Set aside.

> Thread skewer with sausages, onions, apricots, and red pepper. Place on preheated grill, turning frequently until sausages are no longer pink inside. Baste with glaze; cook, turning frequently and continually brushing with glaze, for 1-3 more minutes or until vegetables are tender and sausages are nicely glazed.

> Serves 4.

Nori Wraps

2 bell peppers (red, orange, yellow)

6 shredded carrots

2 Tbsp clarified butter (ghee)

¼ cup unpasteurized soy sauce or coconut aminos

1 tsp dried basil

1 tsp dried oregano

3 cloves of minced garlic

⅔ cup green-fed, raw cheddar cheese or goat cheese

Salt and pepper

Nori

> Sauté minced garlic, peppers, and carrots in the ghee.

> Add herbs, coconut aminos, and cheese.

> Spoon onto a raw nori sheet and wrap.

> Serves 2-4.

salads

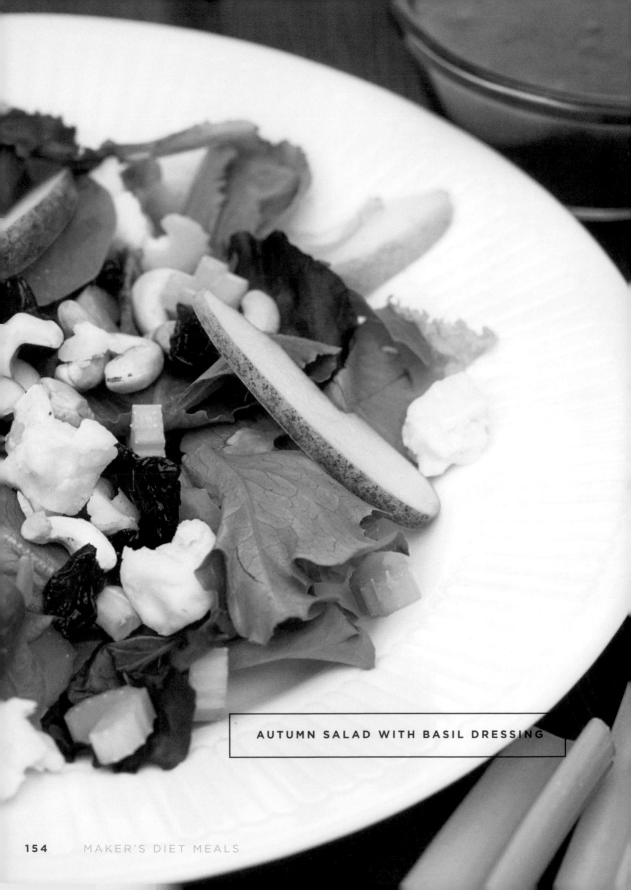

AUTUMN SALAD WITH BASIL DRESSING

Autumn Salad with Basil Dressing

10 oz salad greens

6 oz baby kale

3 oz Italian parsley, trimmed of large stems

1 tart apple, thinly sliced lengthwise

1 green pear, thinly sliced lengthwise

Juice of 1 lemon

⅔ cup tart dried cherries

2 Tbsp hemp seeds

⅔ cup chopped walnuts, soaked and dehydrated or toasted

½ lb green-fed raw cheese or goat cheese

BASIL DRESSING:

¾ cup fresh basil, chopped

¼ cup Italian parsley leaves, no stems

½ cup raw, unheated honey

3 medium-sized garlic cloves

½ cup Terrain Fermented Holy Basil or apple cider vinegar

1 cup almond oil

½ tsp sea salt

Freshly cracked black pepper to taste

> Combine first three ingredients together. Combine the apple and pear slices together in a small bowl and squeeze lemon juice over it.

> Add apple, pear slices, dried cherries, hemp seeds, and walnuts to the salad greens. Crumble the cheese on top just before serving.

> In your food processor, blend basil, parsley, garlic, salt, and pepper until finely ground. Add fermented holy basil or vinegar and honey, pulse several times until well blended. Pour oil in and blend. Refrigerate until ready to use.

> Serves 4-6.

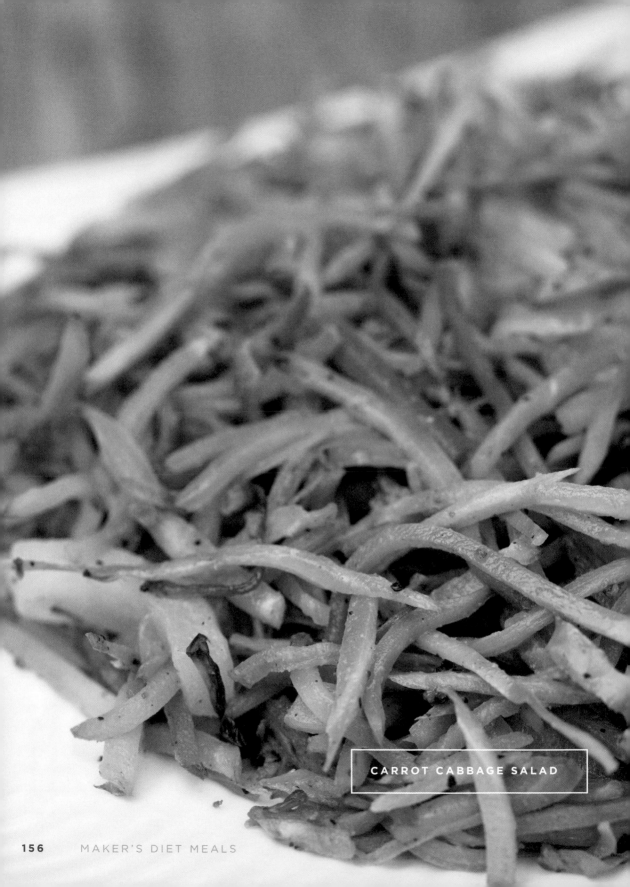

CARROT CABBAGE SALAD

Carrot Cabbage Salad

½ pound whole grain pasta, shredded zucchini, or shredded cucumber

2 or 3 carrots

¼ head of a small cabbage

½ lb of fresh asparagus

1 small cucumber, chopped

¼ of a red onion, thinly sliced

Toasted sesame seeds for garnish

SAUCE:

¼ cup sesame tahini, peanut butter, or almond butter

2 Tbsp unpasteurized soy sauce or coconut aminos

3 Tbsp water

1 Tbsp coconut sugar

1 Tbsp rice vinegar

1 tsp chili paste or a fresh chili, chopped

1 tsp dijon mustard

Pinch of sea salt

Fresh ground pepper

> Cook your pasta according to package directions. Drain and rinse with cold water. After it's drained sufficiently, put it in a bowl with a tablespoon or so of organic extra virgin olive oil and stir it around to prevent it from sticking together. You can prepare the pasta hours before you assemble the salad.

> Cut the cabbage into quarters and remove the core of one of the quarters. Peel the carrots and asparagus. You don't have to peel the asparagus, I just do it because it looks prettier that way.

> Now, set up your food processor and use the disc that has one slit for the cabbage and the disc that has lots of holes for the carrots. You can slice the cabbage thin if you don't have a food processor and grate the carrots. I like to lightly steam the asparagus first or even throw the whole stalk into the boiling pasta water and cook for 2 minutes before the pasta goes in. You can leave them raw if you like.

> Rinse the asparagus and when it's cool, chop into ½ inch pieces. Chop your cucumber up about the same size and thinly slice the red onion and cut the rings into quarters.

> Put all the veggies into the bowl with the pasta and refrigerate until you are ready to eat.

(cont.)

Carrot Cabbage Salad (cont.)

> To make the sauce, put all the ingredients in a little mini food processor or just whisk together in a bowl. I included the peanut butter when I made the sauce, and because it was natural peanut butter it was a little too dry to whisk so I dumped all the ingredients in the little mini processor and let it whirl. It's a wet dressing, not super thick, but it perfectly coats all the pasta and vegetables.

> When you're ready to eat, pour the dressing on the salad and toss it all together. Sprinkle the herbs on top and some toasted sesame seeds.

> Serves 2-4.

TIPS

• There are some perfectly fine gluten free pasta alternatives available. You could also use buckwheat soba noodles. If you want to keep it totally raw, use shredded zucchini or cucumber.

• Be creative with your ingredients. Think chopped red or yellow peppers, broccoli, zucchini, celery, or dark, chopped leafy greens— all would be wonderful in this salad.

• If you don't like tahini just use the peanut or almond butter.

Raw Sprout Salad

1 red onion, sliced

2 cucumbers, washed and sliced

2 cups clover, alfalfa, and broccoli sprouts

1 red bell pepper, sliced

1 yellow bell pepper, sliced

4 heads romaine lettuce, chopped

16 oz pastured chicken, precooked and chopped

2 cups green-fed, raw cheese or goat cheese, shredded

4 avocados, sliced

> Mix ingredients together in salad bowl.
> Serve with homemade Italian dressing (below).
> Serves 4.

Probiotic Infused Italian Dressing

1 cup Terrain Fermented Oregano or apple cider vinegar

3 cloves garlic

1 tsp raw, unheated honey

3 Tbsp mustard

1 Tbsp each of basil, thyme, oregano

1 tsp sea salt

½ tsp black pepper

1 cup extra virgin olive oil

> Blend in a blender and serve over salad.

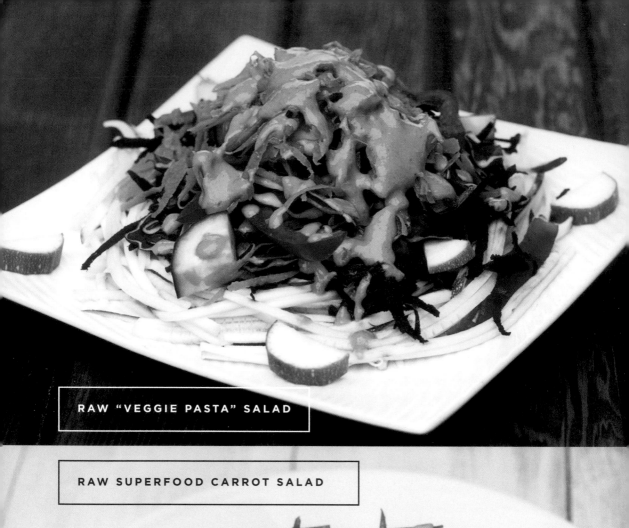

RAW "VEGGIE PASTA" SALAD

RAW SUPERFOOD CARROT SALAD

Raw "Veggie Pasta" Salad

2 spiraled zucchinis

1 orange bell pepper

1 yellow bell pepper

1/2 cup raw, green-fed cheddar, shredded

Raw Italian dressing

DRESSING:

1 cup apple cider vinegar (raw organic)

3 cloves of garlic

1 Tbsp raw, unheated honey

3 Tbsp mustard

1 Tbsp basil, thyme, oregano (each)

1 tsp real salt

½ tsp black pepper

1 cup cold pressed olive oil

> DRESSING: Blend in a blender.
> Toss everything together.
> Chill and eat.
> Serves 2-4.

Raw Superfood Carrot Salad

10 large shredded carrots

1 cup dried goji berries

4 shredded apples

1 cup raw pecans

3 Tbsp dijon mustard

¼ cup fresh squeezed lime juice

¼ cup maple syrup

1 tsp lemon pepper

1 tsp sea salt

> Mix all ingredients together.
> Serve chilled.
> Serves 2.

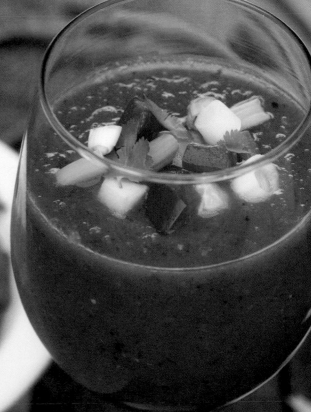

FALL SALAD WITH GREEN DRESSING

GAZPACHO

Fall Salad with Green Dressing

1 head romaine lettuce, chopped

4 cups fresh spinach

2 apples, chopped

1 cup raisins

1 cup raw pecans

1 cup crumbled raw, green-fed cheddar

RAW MAPLE GREEN DRESSING:

7-8 green onions

2-3 large cloves of garlic

1 ¼ cup extra virgin olive oil

⅔ cup maple syrup

1 Tbsp stone ground mustard

½ cup Terrain Fermented Garlic or apple cider vinegar

sea salt and pepper

> SALAD: Mix all ingredients together in bowl.
> DRESSING: Blend all ingredients together in a blender and serve over salad.
> Serves 2-4.

Gazpacho

1 large or 2 medium cucumbers peeled with ¼ cup reserved and chopped for garnish

½ green or red pepper and ½ chopped for garnish

½ chopped medium onion

¼ cup finely chopped scallions for garnish

1 Tbsp chopped parsley

2 tsp chopped chives

3 cups tomato juice

¼ cup extra virgin olive oil

2 Tbsp red wine or balsamic vinegar

1 clove garlic

1 tsp Worcestershire sauce

½ tsp hot pepper sauce (or more to taste)

Sea salt and freshly ground pepper to taste

> Set aside the vegetable garnishes.
> Put everything else in the blender or food processor with half of the tomato juice.
> Puree thoroughly and add the rest of the juice.
> Taste to correct the seasonings.
> Chill and serve with bowls of the chopped garnishes and either Amasai or sheep milk yogurt.
> Serves 2-4.

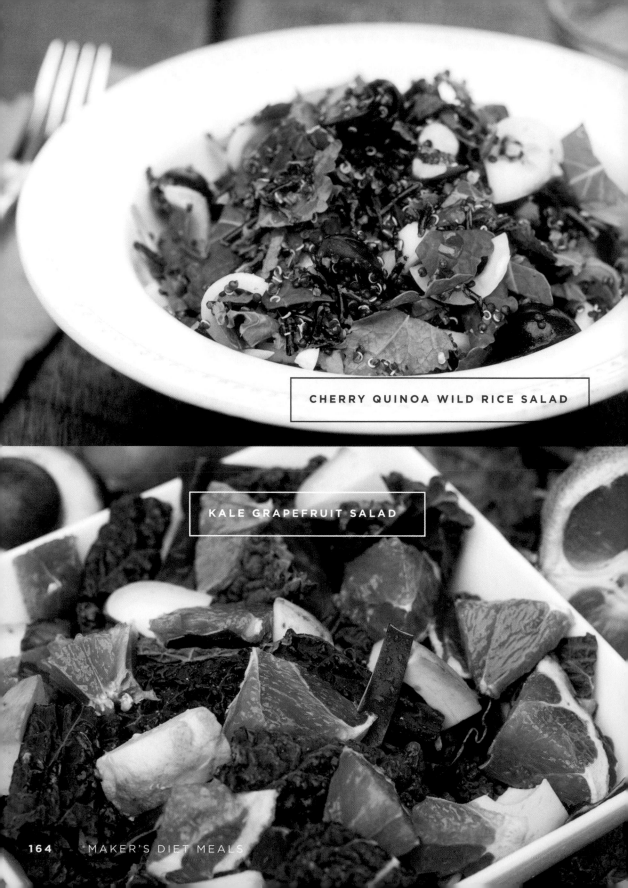

CHERRY QUINOA WILD RICE SALAD

KALE GRAPEFRUIT SALAD

Cherry Quinoa Wild Rice Salad

2 cups pitted and halved dark red cherries

2 cups cooked red quinoa

½ cup wild rice

1 cup chopped raw kale

½ cup chopped celery

½ cup chopped raw or sprouted nuts (almonds, cashews, or pecans)

Sea salt and pepper to taste

¼ cup extra virgin olive oil

¼ cup Terrain Fermented Kombucha or apple cider vinegar

1 tsp stone ground or dijon mustard

1 clove minced garlic

> Soak quinoa at least 15 minutes to remove the bitter coating.

> Cook the wild rice in 3 cups of water for 15 minutes.

> Drain the quinoa and add it to the wild rice.

> Continue to cook for 15 minutes more just until the quinoa is done. It should be al dente, not mushy.

> Drain in a colander.

> Combine the quinoa and wild rice mixture, the vegetables, cherries, and nuts in a large bowl.

> Whisk together the oil, vinegar, mustard, garlic, salt, and pepper and pour over the salad.

> Feel free to be creative with ingredients. Try crisp chunks of apples, dried cherries, cranberries or any veggies you have on hand.

> This would be really good with small chunks of raw cheddar.

> Serves 4.

Kale Grapefruit Salad

3 cups lacinto kale

1 grapefruit, peeled and cut

1 cup purple cabbage

½ avocado, sliced

> Place all ingredients in bowl.

> Squeeze fresh lemon over the top with black pepper.

> Serves 2-4.

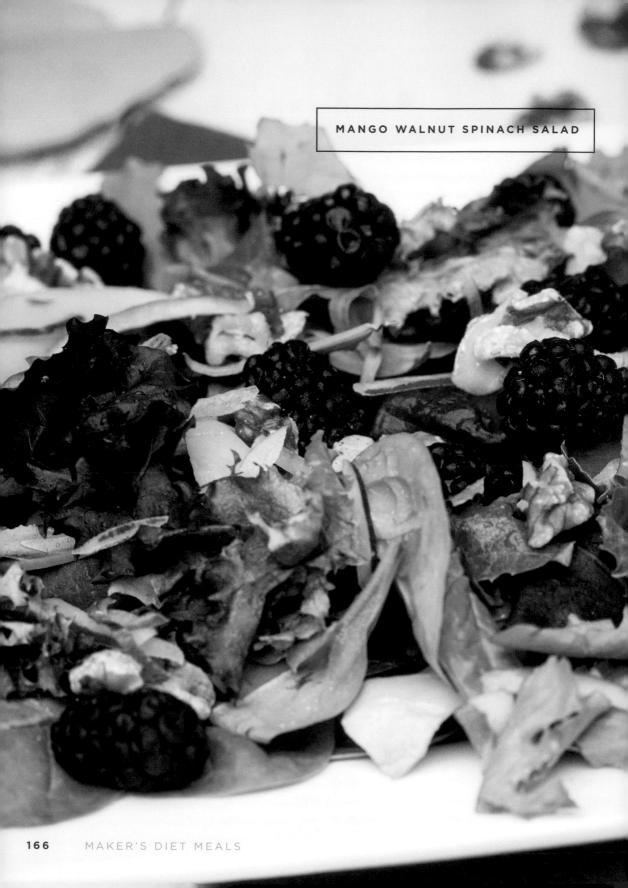

MANGO WALNUT SPINACH SALAD

Mango Walnut Spinach Salad

½ pound baby spinach

2 cups baby kale (optional)

1 lb mixed spring salad mix

1 small red onion, sliced thin

2 mangos, peeled, seeded and cut into strips

1 cup fresh blackberries

½ cup rough chopped walnuts, soaked and dehydrated or toasted

MANGO DRESSING:

2 ripe mangos, peeled, seeded, and pureed in blender to make ⅓ cup

2 Tbsp fresh squeezed orange juice

1 Tbsp fresh squeezed lime juice

2 Tbsp Terrain Fermented Kombucha or apple cider vinegar

2 cloves garlic, minced

2 Tbsp extra virgin olive oil

1 Tbsp raw, unheated honey

1 tsp sea salt

2 Tbsp fresh parsley, chopped

> Soak and dehydrate or toast walnuts in a small skillet over medium-high heat for 3-4 minutes until toasted and lightly browned. Place cooled walnuts and rest of salad ingredients in salad bowl and toss. Serve with Mango Dressing.

> MANGO DRESSING: Puree mango and measure ⅓ cup. Add rest of the ingredients except chopped parsley to blender and blend until well mixed. Pour into bowl and add parsley.

> Serves 6.

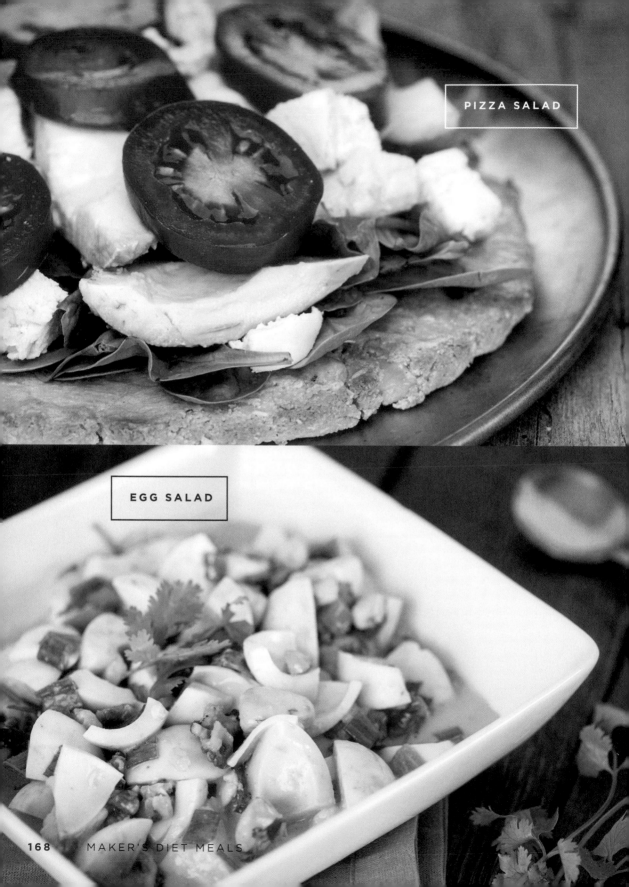

PIZZA SALAD

EGG SALAD

Pizza Salad

CRUST:

3 cups almond flour

3 pastured eggs

1 tsp sea salt

½ cup green-fed raw cheddar cheese or goat cheese

TOPPINGS:

2 Tbsp coconut oil mayonnaise (see recipe on page 187)

2 cups romaine, chopped

1 tomato, sliced

1 avocado, sliced

4 oz pastured chicken, chopped

Grass-fed beef summer sausage (optional)

CRUST:
> Mix all ingredients together.
> Roll out onto a stoneware pan and bake at 350 for 15-20 minutes.

TOPPINGS:
> Spread mayo over crust.
> Add remaining toppings.
> Serve!
> Serves 4.

Egg Salad

5 hard boiled pastured eggs

½ cup coconut oil mayonnaise (see recipe on page 187)

¼ cup celery

¼ cup sprouted pecans

¼ cup raisins

Sea salt and pepper

> Chop eggs, celery, and pecans.
> Combine all ingredients together.
> Serve chilled.
> Serves 2.

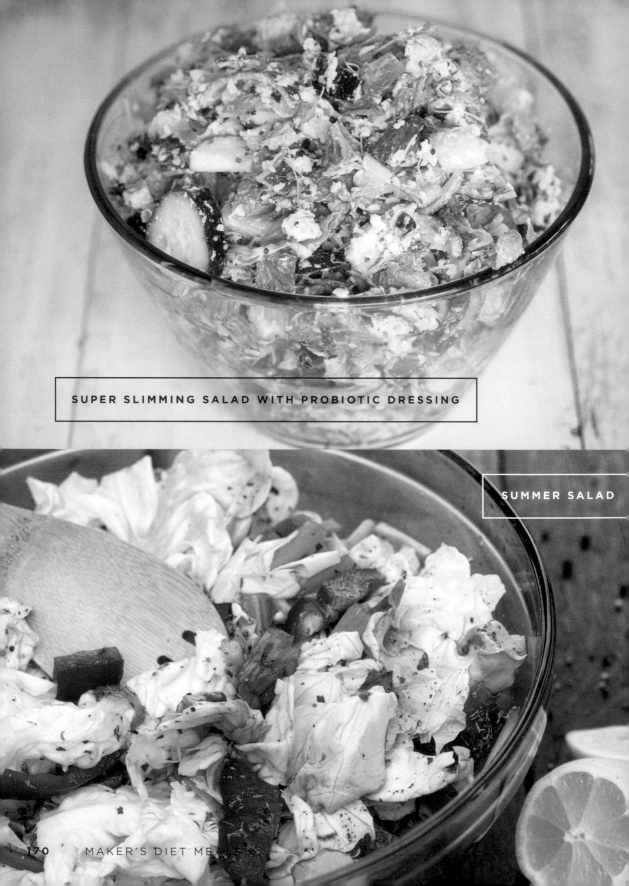

SUPER SLIMMING SALAD WITH PROBIOTIC DRESSING

SUMMER SALAD

Super Slimming Salad with Probiotic Dressing

2 cups sprouts (clover, broccoli, or alfalfa)

2 heads butter leaf lettuce

4 cups baby kale

2 cups spinach

2 cups cucumber (seeded and chopped)

1 red onion chopped (chop it right before adding to salad)

2 cups shredded raw, green-fed harvarti cheese

1 cup ground chia seeds

Probiotic ranch dressing

DRESSING:

8 oz Amasai or sheep milk yogurt

1 cup homemade mayonnaise (see recipe on page 187)

1 Tbsp dried basil

1 tsp dried dill weed

3 garlic cloves, minced

> Mix all ingredients in a bowl.
> Serve chilled.
> Serves 4.

DRESSING:
> Whisk together all ingredients.

Summer Salad

3 heads romaine lettuce

2 yellow and red bell peppers, sliced

1 cucumber, diced

1 red onion, sliced

6 green onions, chopped

> Throw all ingredients together in large bowl.
> Pour lemon juice and apple cider vinegar over salad.
> Serves 4-6.

Cheesy, Lemony, Quinoa and Avocado Salad

2 cups cooked quinoa

4 ripe avocados, peeled and cubed

Zest of 2 lemons and their juice

¼ cup extra virgin olive oil

½ cup red onion, finely chopped

½ cup green-fed, raw cheese or goat cheese, chunked

½ cup raw or sprouted nuts

> Soak quinoa for at least 15 minutes to remove the bitter coating.

> Cook in 3 cups water until al dente, not mushy.

> Drain but don't rinse. Let quinoa cool. This step can be done well in advance.

> Remove the zest from the lemons (you can lightly freeze them to make this easier) and squeeze out all the juice.

> Whisk the lemon juice and the olive oil together.

> Combine all the ingredients in a large bowl and mix gently. Add salt and pepper to taste.

> Some fresh, minced garlic and chopped parsley would take this over the top!

> Serves 8.

Tuscan Salmon Salad

8 cups spring mix salad greens

6 hard boiled pastured eggs, quartered

1 lb asparagus, trimmed

1 ½ Tbsp extra virgin olive oil

1 ½ cups cherry tomatoes, halved

12-oz jar of artichoke hearts, well drained

⅓ cup pitted black olives

1 small red onion, thinly sliced

12 oz honey glazed cooked salmon (recipe below)

1 Tbsp fresh basil, thinly sliced

1 tsp fresh thyme, chopped

1 tsp fresh oregano, chopped

Sea salt and fresh pepper to taste

HONEY DIJON SALMON:

2 Tbsp raw, unheated honey

1 Tbsp balsamic vinegar

2 Tbsp dijon mustard

2 Tbsp unpasteurized soy sauce or coconut aminos

2 Tbsp olive oil

Sea salt and freshly ground black pepper

2 wild-caught salmon fillets

> In medium saucepan, bring salted water to a boil. Add asparagus and cook for about 2 minutes. Immediately drain asparagus and plunge in ice water to stop the cooking. Heat a skillet over medium-high heat until hot but not smoking.

> In medium bowl, add greens, tomatoes, asparagus, artichokes, black olives, and red onions. Add quartered eggs, fresh basil, thyme, and oregano over salad. With a fork, gently flake the cooled salmon into large chunks. Add Tuscan Salad Dressing.

> Using the same hot skillet used to cook the asparagus, heat skillet to medium heat. Brush salmon with olive oil and season with salt and pepper to taste. Coat the flesh of the salmon fillets with the honey mixture. When skillet is hot again, sauté for 6-8 minutes to medium doneness, turning once after five minutes, until fish flakes easily.

> Squeeze lemon juice over salmon. Allow to cool.

(cont.)

TUSCAN SALAD DRESSING:

1 garlic clove, minced

Liquid drained from the artichokes

1 tsp fresh lemon juice

1 Tbsp balsamic vinegar

3 Tbsp fresh basil, minced

1 tsp fresh thyme, chopped

¼ tsp dried dill

¼ tsp red pepper flakes

¼ cup grated aged green-fed, raw Havarti cheese

½ cup extra virgin olive oil

> Add all ingredients except oil in food processor and pulse several times until well blended and garlic is chopped fine. While food processor is still running, add olive oil slowly until dressing is creamy and well blended.

> Serves 8

Grilled Salad

8 oz romaine lettuce, chopped

8 oz spring mix salad greens

4 oz baby kale

3 Roma tomatoes, cut in half lengthwise

2 avocados, pitted and cut into 8 strips each

1 red onion, cut into ½ inch chunks

1 red pepper, cut into ¾ inch strips

1 yellow pepper, cut into ¾ inch strips

1 ripe mango, peeled, deseeded, and cut into long strips about ½ inch thick

2 boneless, skinless pasture-raised grilled chicken breasts sliced thin

> Combine ingredients in large salad bowl and drizzle dressing.

DRESSING:

¼ cup balsamic vinegar

1 lg. garlic clove, finely minced

3 tsp raw, unheated honey

1 tsp dijon mustard

¾ cup olive oil

Sea salt and pepper to taste

> Put all ingredients in a covered jar and shake well.

> Serves 4-6.

Steak Salad with Chipotle Aioli

STEAK:

2 lbs of grass-fed beef tenderloin

½ cup extra virgin olive oil

¼ cup unpasteurized soy sauce or coconut aminos

¼ cup Worcestershire sauce

¼ cup pineapple juice

2 Tbsp minced garlic cloves

1 Tbsp dry mustard

1 tsp dried basil

½ tsp onion powder

> In a medium-sized bowl, whisk all ingredients together. Put steak in a glass baking dish or ziplock plastic, and add marinade. Refrigerate for at least 4 hours but no longer than 10 hours. Grill or sauté steak.

> Put steak on bed of salad and add aioli on top.

> Serves 4-6.

AIOLI:

1 cup homemade mayonnaise (see recipe on page 187)

¼ cup dijon mustard

1 garlic clove, minced

⅛ tsp onion powder

2 Tbsp white wine vinegar

1 Tbsp minced chipotle chilies with adobo sauce

½ tsp fresh lemon juice

> Whisk all ingredients together to blend well. Cover and put in refrigerator, at least 1 hour before serving.

Spinach Salad with Cherries

SALAD:

4 cups baby spinach

1 tart apple, sliced into thin slices

Juice from 1 lemon

2 Tbsp sunflower seeds

¼ cup pumpkin seeds, toasted

½ cup dried cherries

½ cup sliced raw mushrooms

¼ cup shaved aged green-fed, raw Havarti cheese

> Slice apples and squeeze lemon juice over slices. Toss to coat all slices. Slice mushrooms and add to spinach. Add sliced apples, shaved cheese, cooled seeds, and cherries. Serve with the cherry vinaigrette.

CHERRY VINAIGRETTE:

½ cup frozen cherries, thawed

¼ cup white balsamic vinegar

1 tsp dijon mustard

1 cup almond oil

3 Tbsp raw, unheated honey

2 Tbsp thinly sliced green onions

Sea salt and freshly ground pepper to taste

> Put thawed cherries (with their juice) in food processor. Pulse until cherries are pureed. Add balsamic vinegar, honey, oil, and mustard to cherries and blend again. Add the sliced green onions. Season with salt and pepper.

> Serves 4.

Southwest Avocado Salad

CHICKEN:

2 large pasture-raised chicken breasts, slightly flattened

2 Tbsp extra virgin olive oil

Sea salt and pepper to season

1 tsp smoked paprika

1 tsp chili powder

½ tsp granulated garlic

½ tsp onion powder

> Mix all dry ingredients together well. Rub both sides of chicken breasts with olive oil and spice mixture. Put pan or grill at medium-high heat. Add chicken breasts to pan or grill and cook for about 10-12 minutes.

SALAD:

1 bunch of bibb lettuce, washed, dried and torn into bite sized pieces

1 head romaine lettuce, washed, dried and torn into bite sized pieces

1 red bell pepper, diced

14.5 oz can black beans, rinsed and drained well

1 cup frozen corn, thawed

1 cup cherry tomatoes, halved

4 green onions, thin sliced

¼ cup cilantro leaves, rough chopped

Juice of 1 lemon

> Combine all ingredients in large platter. Toss to combine. Place sliced chicken breasts on top of greens and drizzle avocado dressing over the chicken. Place more dressing at the table.

AVOCADO SALAD DRESSING:

1 large ripe avocado, peeled and pitted

1 Tbsp fresh lemon juice

1 garlic clove, minced

½ cup mayonnaise

¼ cup olive oil

¼ tsp cayenne pepper

½ tsp sea salt

1 Tbsp green onions, chopped

1 Tbsp fresh cilantro, chopped

¼ cup plain Amasai or sheep milk yogurt

> In a food processor or blender, blend all ingredients except the green onions and cilantro until creamy. Add green onions and cilantro and pulse or blend quickly to mix well, but still see bits of the cilantro.

> Serves 6.

side dishes

CHUNKY TOMATO SALSA

Chunky Tomato Salsa

3 garden fresh tomatoes, diced

⅔ cup fresh cilantro

1 diced jalapeno pepper

¼ cup red onion, diced

Fresh juice from two fresh limes

Fresh juice from half an orange

Sea salt and pepper to taste

> Mix all ingredients together.
> Serve with fresh guacamole and chicken.
> Serves 6.

Cauliflower "Rice"

4 heads cauliflower

1 tsp sea salt

½ cup unpasteurized soy sauce or coconut aminos

> With a cheese grater, grate cauliflower.
> Mix in salt and coconut aminos and put in a large glass bowl and bake at 350 for 20-30 minutes.
> Serves 6.

Sautéed Asian Broccoli

9-oz package broccoli florets

2-3 Tbsp extra virgin olive oil

1 small sweet onion, rough chopped

1 Tbsp unpasteurized soy sauce or coconut aminos

1 tsp garlic, minced

1 tsp sea salt

1 Tbsp sesame tahini

Black pepper to taste

> Sauté broccoli florets and onion in olive oil for about 4 minutes over medium heat or until it is starting to soften. Add garlic, sea salt, and black pepper and continue to sauté for 1 minute. Add tahini and soy sauce, stir well, and cook for one minute. Serve immediately.
> Serves 4.

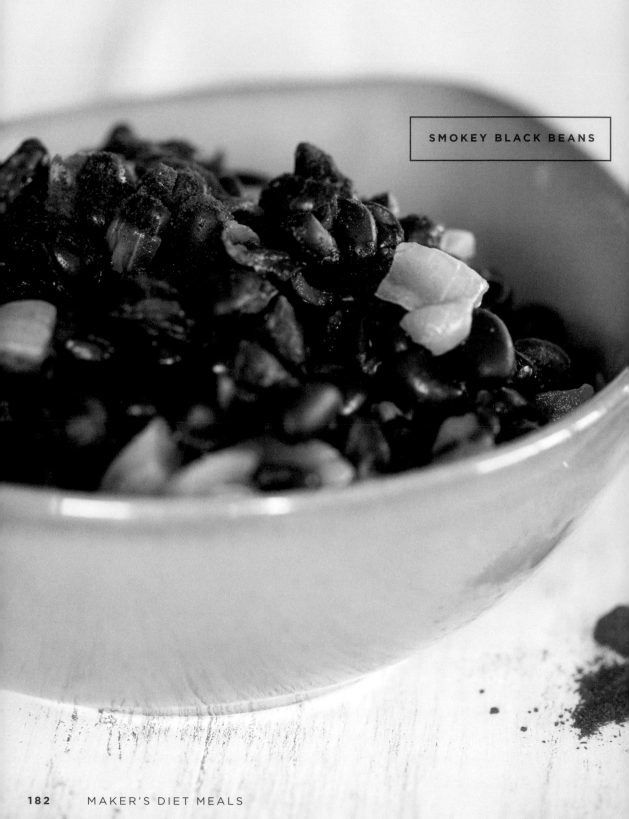

SMOKEY BLACK BEANS

Smokey Black Beans

1 large yellow onion, chopped (vidalia or another sweet onion if available)

2 Tbsp coconut oil

2 cloves garlic, chopped

2 cans black beans

1 cup chicken or vegetable broth

1 to 3 tsp smoked hot paprika

1 avocado, cut into chunks

½ cup plain Amasai

2 fresh limes

> Heat the oil over medium heat in a large pan.

> Add the onions and garlic and sauté until the onion is soft but not brown, about 5-7 minutes.

> Add the smoked paprika and stir it around into the onions. The smell is heavenly!

> Now add your black beans and stir it all together and add chicken broth so it doesn't stick to the bottom of the pan. Cook for about 10 minutes or so and if it starts to get dry, go ahead and add more chicken broth. You want it wet but not soupy.

> While the beans are cooking, peel and chop an avocado and quarter the two limes.

> Serve in bowls with the avocado, limes, and Amasai as a garnish.

> Smoked paprika is available both hot and sweet (meaning not hot). The sweet is just as delicious if you don't like spicy.

> Serves 2 as a meal, 3 or 4 as a side dish

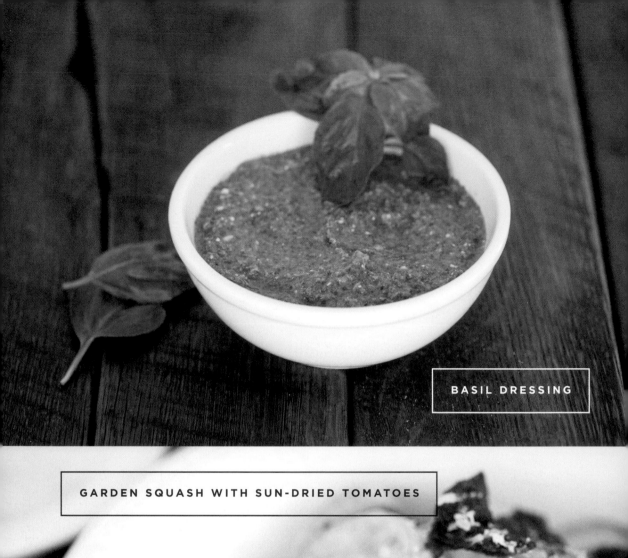

BASIL DRESSING

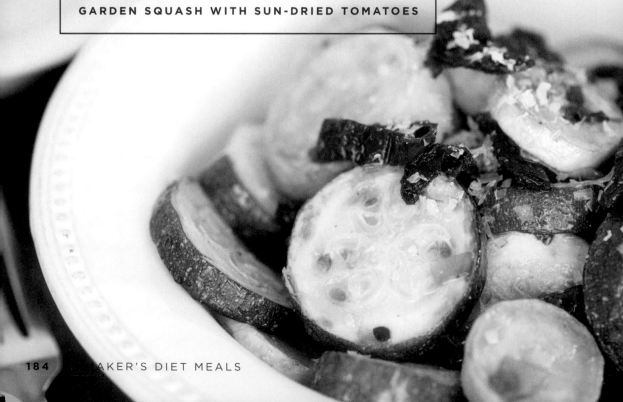

GARDEN SQUASH WITH SUN-DRIED TOMATOES

Basil Dressing

¾ cup fresh basil, chopped

¼ cup Italian parsley leaves, no stems

½ cup raw, unheated honey

3 medium-sized garlic cloves

½ cup apple cider vinegar

1 cup organic grapeseed oil

½ tsp sea salt

Freshly cracked black pepper to taste

> In your food processor, using the medal blade, blend basil, parsley, garlic, salt, and pepper until finely ground.
> Add vinegar and honey, pulse several times until well blended.
> Pour oil in through the small feed tube so that it pours very slowly and in a steady stream.
> Blend until all the oil is incorporated and everything is blended well.
> Refrigerate until ready to use.

Garden Squash with Sun-Dried Tomatoes

1 6-oz jar sun-dried tomatoes with herbs, undrained

4 medium-sized yellow squash

4 medium-sized zucchini

2 shallots, finely diced

2 Tbsp fresh basil, sliced thin

Sea salt and pepper to taste

> Slice zucchini and yellow squash into ¼ inch slices. Add your reserved oil to a medium skillet. Add the diced shallots, and both squashes. Sauté until squash is becoming soft and lightly browned over medium-high heat.
> Add reserved sun-dried tomatoes strips and basil. Toss gently to mix. Serve immediately.
> Serves 6.

ROASTED CAULIFLOWER WITH CHILI LIME BUTTER

Roasted Cauliflower
with Chili Lime Butter

1 head of cauliflower

2-3 cloves of garlic, peeled and minced

2 Tbsp fresh squeezed lemon juice

Coarse salt and freshly ground black pepper

1 tsp chili powder

¼ cup olive oil

¼ cup aged green-fed, raw Havarti cheese

Chili lime butter (see recipe)

CHILE LIME BUTTER:

½ stick (¼ cup) unsalted grass-fed butter, softened

1 Tbsp finely chopped shallot

1 tsp finely grated fresh lime zest

1 tsp fresh lime juice

½ tsp adobo sauce from canned chipotle peppers with adobo sauce

> Cut cauliflower into florets and put in a single layer in an oven-proof baking dish. Toss in the garlic. Sprinkle lemon juice over cauliflower and drizzle each piece with the olive oil. Sprinkle with salt and pepper and the chili powder.

> Bake at 400 degrees uncovered for 25-30 minutes.

> Remove from oven and sprinkle generously with cheese. Drizzle with the chili lime butter. Serve immediately.

> CHILI LIME BUTTER: In a small saucepan, mix all ingredients together over medium-low heat and cook just until the butter is melted.

> Serves 4.

GRILLED CABBAGE

COCONUT OIL MAYO

Grilled Cabbage

1 head green cabbage

½ cup melted grass-fed butter

1 tsp black pepper

> Preheat an outdoor grill for medium-high heat.
> Slice the top off of the head of cabbage so that it will sit flat with the cored side up.
> Slice cabbage into 5 large pieces.
> Season with butter and pepper.
> Wrap tightly with foil.
> Place wrapped cabbage down directly on the grill.
> Let cook for 25-30 minutes, or until tender and serve.
> Serves 4.

Coconut Oil Mayo

3 pastured egg yolks, room temperature

1 tsp mustard

1 ½ tsp fresh lemon juice

2 Tbsp cultured whey

¾ cup coconut oil (make sure it's melted all the way)

Pinch of sea salt and black pepper

> In food processor or high-speed blender, blend all ingredients except oil at very low power. Slowly drizzle in oil. Let that combine for at least a minute! Scoop into container and screw the lid on very tightly. Leave mayonnaise out for 7 hours before refrigerating. Mayonnaise will keep in fridge for several months.

CRUSTLESS SPINACH QUICHE

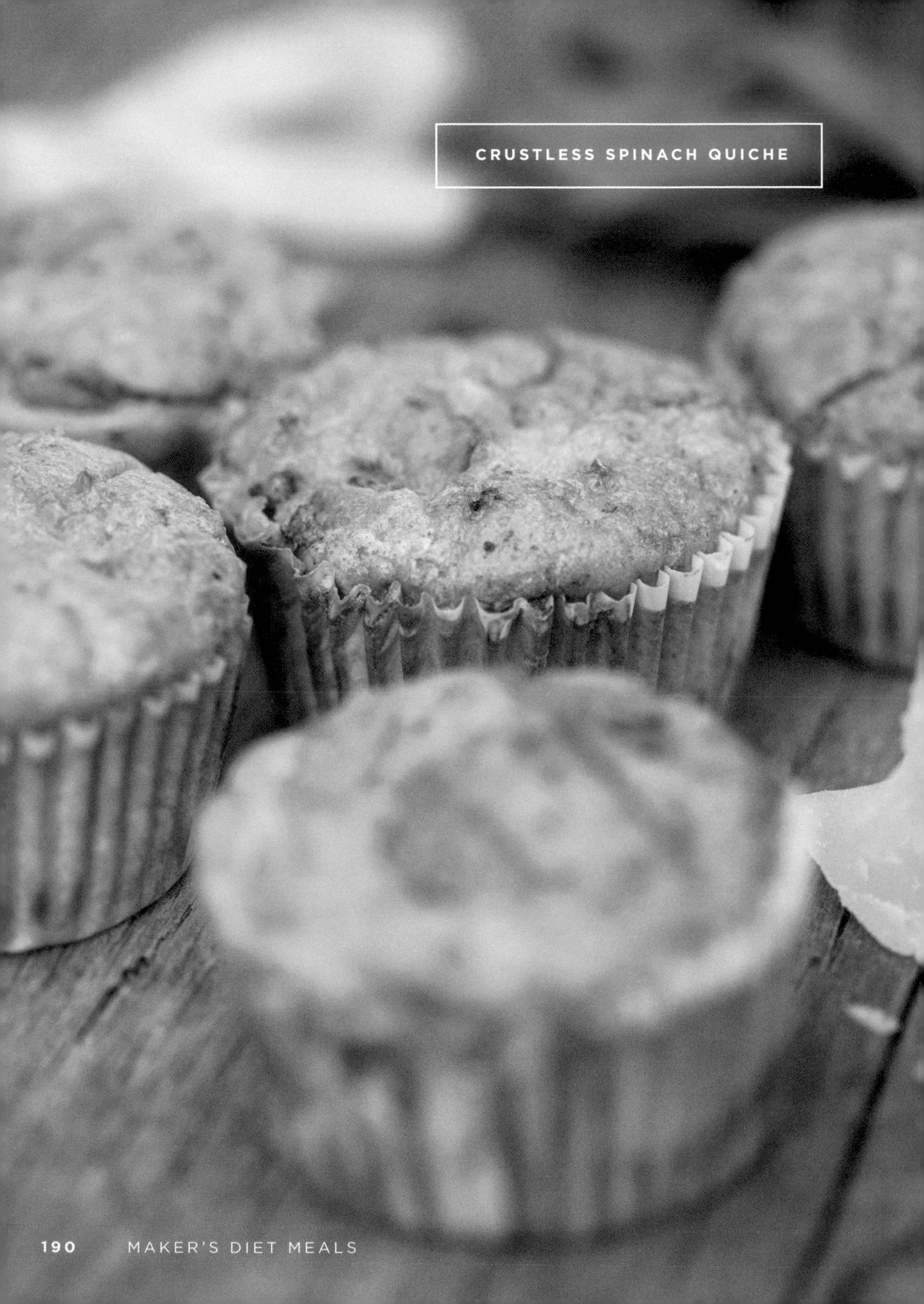

Crustless Spinach Quiche

4 pastured eggs

¼ cup Amasai or sheep milk yogurt

½ tsp sea salt

⅔ cup frozen spinach

2 cloves of garlic

½ cup onion, chopped

⅓ cup coconut flour

½ tsp baking powder

Black pepper to taste

> Blend eggs, Amasai, salt, spinach, garlic, and onion together in a high-speed blender.

> Add coconut flour and baking powder and blend.

> Grease muffin tin with coconut oil or line it with muffin cups.

> Drop batter in by heaping tablespoons at a time.

> Sprinkle with black pepper.

> Serves 4.

Coconut Lime Quinoa

1 cup quinoa

½ cup coconut milk

½ cup chicken broth

½ tsp sea salt

2 Tbsp lime juice, divided

Zest of 2 limes

2 Tbsp fresh cilantro leaves, chopped

> Rinse quinoa in cool water in a very fine sieve. Add quinoa, coconut milk, 1 Tbsp lime juice, and chicken broth in saucepan and bring to a boil. When mixture comes to a boil, lower heat and cover. Cook for about 10-15 minutes until liquid is absorbed and quinoa is fully cooked. Turn off burner and let stand, covered, for 5 minutes.

> Fluff quinoa with a fork and add the cilantro, lime zest, and 1 tablespoon lime juice.

> Serves 4.

Roasted Avocado and Southwest Quinoa

4 avocados, halved

2 Tbsp lemon juice

2 Tbsp extra virgin olive oil

Sea salt and pepper

SOUTHWEST QUINOA

1 cup quinoa

2 cups chicken broth

½ tsp whole cumin

8 oz black beans, strained

8 oz can whole kernel corn, drained

½ Tbsp chili powder

2 Roma tomatoes, diced

3 Tbsp cilantro, chopped fine

½ cup red onion, diced

1 Tbsp garlic, minced

2 Tbsp Italian parsley, finely chopped

1 lime

> Prepare quinoa using the 2 cups of chicken broth and 1 cup quinoa.

> Cut avocado into quarters, drizzle with a little olive oil, lemon juice, and season generously with salt and pepper. Bake at 400 for 15 minutes.

> In bowl mix black beans, chili powder, Roma tomatoes, cilantro, red onions, garlic, parsley, cumin, and lime juice. Add quinoa to the bowl and mix.

> Serves 4

Pesto Quinoa

1 cup vegetable broth

½ cup quinoa

1 8-oz jar of unsulfured sun-dried tomatoes

2 cups loosely packed fresh basil

2 cloves garlic

¼ cup walnuts or pine nuts

¼ cup olive oil

¼ cup grated aged green-fed, raw cheese

> Add quinoa to vegetable broth and bring to a boil. When mixture comes to a boil, reduce heat, cover, and cook for 10-15 minutes.

> To make pesto, blend all remaining ingredients for pesto in food processor until creamy.

> Add ⅓ cup tomato pesto to the cooked quinoa.

> Makes about 1 ½ cups of quinoa.